D1103851

Play Therapy Interventions
to Enhance Resilience

CREATIVE ARTS AND PLAY THERAPY

Cathy A. Malchiodi and David A. Crenshaw, Series Editors

This series highlights action-oriented therapeutic approaches that utilize art, play, music, dance/movement, drama, and related modalities. Emphasizing current best practices and research, experienced practitioners show how creative arts and play therapies can be integrated into overall treatment for individuals of all ages. Books in the series provide richly illustrated guidelines and techniques for addressing trauma, attachment problems, and other psychological difficulties, as well as for supporting resilience and self-regulation.

Creative Arts and Play Therapy for Attachment Problems
Cathy A. Malchiodi and David A. Crenshaw, Editors

Play Therapy: A Comprehensive Guide to Theory and Practice
David A. Crenshaw and Anne L. Stewart, Editors

Creative Interventions with Traumatized Children,
Second Edition
Cathy A. Malchiodi, Editor

Music Therapy Handbook
Barbara L. Wheeler, Editor

Play Therapy Interventions to Enhance Resilience
David A. Crenshaw, Robert Brooks, and Sam Goldstein, Editors

Play Therapy
Interventions to
Enhance Resilience

edited by
David A. Crenshaw
Robert Brooks
Sam Goldstein

THE GUILFORD PRESS
New York   London

Library of Congress Cataloging-in-Publication Data

Play therapy interventions to enhance resilience / edited by David A. Crenshaw,
Robert Brooks, Sam Goldstein.
    p. ; cm. — (Creative arts and play therapy)
  Includes bibliographical references and index.
  ISBN 978-1-4625-2046-6 (hardcover : alk. paper)
  I. Crenshaw, David A. editor.   II. Brooks, Robert B., editor.   III. Goldstein,
Sam, 1952– , editor.   IV. Series: Creative arts and play therapy.
  [DNLM: 1. Play Therapy—methods.   2. Child.   3. Mental Disorders—
therapy.   4. Resilience, Psychological.   WS 350.4]
  RJ505.P6
  618.92891653—dc23
                                                            2014039364

About the Editors

David A. Crenshaw, PhD, ABPP, RPT-S, is Clinical Director of the Children's Home of Poughkeepsie, New York. A Fellow of the American Psychological Association and of its Division of Clinical Child and Adolescent Psychology, he is past president of the Hudson Valley Psychological Association, which honored him with its Lifetime Achievement Award, and of the New York Association for Play Therapy. Dr. Crenshaw served on the editorial board of the *International Journal of Play Therapy*; taught graduate play therapy courses at Johns Hopkins University; and has published widely on child therapy, child abuse and trauma, and resilience in children. His books include *Creative Arts and Play Therapy for Attachment Problems* (coedited with Cathy A. Malchiodi) and *Play Therapy: A Comprehensive Guide to Theory and Practice* (coedited with Anne L. Stewart).

Robert Brooks, PhD, ABPP, is Assistant Clinical Professor of Psychology in the Department of Psychiatry at Harvard Medical School and former Director of the Department of Psychology at McLean Hospital. He has lectured nationally and internationally and written extensively about such topics as resilience, psychotherapy, and positive school and work environments. Dr. Brooks has coauthored and coedited numerous books with Sam Goldstein, including *Handbook of Resilience in Children, Second Edition*; *Raising Resilient Children*; and *The Power of Resilience*. He has received numerous awards in recognition of his work on behalf of children and their families, especially in the area of resilience.

Sam Goldstein, PhD, is Assistant Clinical Instructor in the Department of Psychiatry at the University of Utah School of Medicine and on staff at the University Neuropsychiatric Institute. He is also Clinical Director of the Neurology, Learning, and Behavior Center in Salt Lake City. Dr. Goldstein is Editor-in-Chief of the *Journal of Attention Disorders* and serves on the editorial boards of six journals He is author or editor of more than 50 books and 100 scholarly publications, as well as several psychological tests. Dr. Goldstein has lectured to thousands of professionals and the lay public in the United States, South America, Asia, Australia, and Europe.

Contributors

Steven Baron, PsyD, West Hempstead Union Free School District, West Hempstead, New York; private practice, Massapequa, New York

Robert Brooks, PhD, Department of Psychiatry, McLean Hospital, Harvard Medical School, Boston, Massachusetts; private practice, Needham, Massachusetts

Suzanne Brooks, PsyD, Weston Public Schools, Weston, Massachusetts

Stephanie Carnes, LMSW, Children's Home of Poughkeepsie, Poughkeepsie, New York

David A. Crenshaw, PhD, ABPP, RPT-S, Children's Home of Poughkeepsie, Poughkeepsie, New York

Eliana Gil, PhD, LMFT, RPT-S, ATR, Gil Institute for Trauma Recovery and Education, Fairfax, Virginia

Sam Goldstein, PhD, Department of Psychiatry, University of Utah School of Medicine, Salt Lake City, Utah

Jillian E. Kelly, LCSW, Urban Health Plan, Inc., Bronx, New York

Cathy A. Malchiodi, Ph.D., ATR-BC, LPAT, LPCC, REAT, Division of Expressive Therapies, Lesley University, Cambridge, Massachusetts; Trauma-Informed Practices and Expressive Arts Therapy Institute, Louisville, Kentucky

Claudio Mochi, RP, RPT-S, Italian Association for Play Therapy and International Academy for Play Therapy and Psychosocial Studies, Rome, Italy

John W. Seymour, PhD, LMFT, RPT-S, Department of Counseling and Student Personnel, Minnesota State University, Mankato, Minnesota

Cherie L. Spehar, LCSW, CTC-S, RPT-S, Smiling Spirit Pathways, Apex, North Carolina

Risë VanFleet, PhD, RPT-S, CDBC, Playful Pooch Program, Family Enhancement and Play Therapy Center, Boiling Springs, Pennsylvania

Preface

The human capacity for burden is like bamboo—far more flexible than you'd ever believe at first glance.
—JODI PICOULT, *My Sister's Keeper*

The growth of a particular topic such as resilience is marked not only by the peer-reviewed scientific literature published about it each year but also by the comprehensive, scientific, and clinical volumes published about it. Resilience has grown as a field to the point at which texts related to specific issues within the field (e.g., assessment and specialized treatment) are now appearing. As the recognition of this important phenomenon in mental health, medicine, and education has increased, risks for the promotion of biased or ineffective treatment strategies have increased in parallel. The need for a carefully crafted guide to resilience-based treatment has become paramount. We have created this volume to serve as such a guide for clinicians.

This book has its roots not only in the research and writings of seminal thinkers and practitioners in the field of resilience over the past four decades but also in the courage of children who have motivated the highly regarded authors and dedicated clinicians whose chapters appear within. Of the three coeditors, Robert Brooks and Sam Goldstein are leaders and prolific authors in the field of child resilience; David A. Crenshaw continues, after more than 45 years, his direct work with at-risk youth, stubbornly refusing to give up no matter the obstacles. He constantly looks for those "islands of competence" so aptly described long ago by Robert Brooks.

The contributors to this volume all share a common faith in children. They find redeemable qualities in those youngsters whose difficulties may have discouraged other helpers, sometimes (although relatively rarely) including their own parents and teachers. In our experience, however, most parents and teachers do the best they can to guide children and to turn around the lives of young people who have taken a destructive path; we have known a significant number of parents and teachers who are nothing short of heroic. Sometimes young people go into a downward spiral in spite of the best efforts of those who love and guide them. Often these youth, believing they are unworthy of the care and help they receive, are gold-medal masters in discouraging those who befriend and try to help them. The contributors to this volume share a passionate belief that "resilient mindsets" and the presence of one or more "charismatic adults," as so beautifully described in the opening chapter by Brooks and Goldstein, can turn around the lives of deeply troubled youth.

Another compelling reason for producing this book is the power of the natural properties of play, especially therapeutic play, to facilitate resilience. The ways in which play not only promotes healthy cognitive, emotional, and social development but also develops resilience in children are described in depth by John W. Seymour, a noted play therapist and scholar on resilience, in Chapter 2. Creative strategies involving metaphors and storytelling are detailed by Robert and Suzanne Brooks in Chapter 3, along with rich case examples illustrating how these interventions amplify resilience. Chapter 4, by David A. Crenshaw and Jillian E. Kelly, poignantly illustrates play therapy techniques that proved useful in the treatment of a heroic and inspiring child whose life tragically ended after she made remarkable gains in therapy. In Chapter 5, Eliana Gil, a renowned play therapist and prolific author, tells the story of another courageous child and mother who rose above the most horrific adversity in their treatment with her. Some of the play therapy interventions described in this chapter will inspire and inform readers who are confronted with severe cases of child trauma in their own practices. In Chapter 6, another internationally known therapist and prolific author, Cathy A. Malchiodi, outlines the use of play and art therapy strategies in a compelling case of child trauma.

In Chapter 7, Steven Baron, who has worked as a school psychologist for nearly three decades, describes the use of strength-based interventions to augment resilience in a very different setting, the public school system; he includes a range of fascinating vignettes. Chapter 8, by Risë VanFleet and Claudio Mochi (widely acclaimed not only as play therapists but also for their work in international disasters), describes the use of play therapy interventions in the aftermath of a major disaster. This chapter is of great current relevance to many in child mental health, because, unfortunately, there has been no shortage of mass disasters in recent years. Chapter 9, by Stephanie Carnes and David A. Crenshaw, also addresses a high-risk population where many in the field might not expect to find "islands of competence." The chapter describes a group play therapy intervention with high-risk adolescent mothers and their babies to promote mother–infant attachment and resilience. Chapter 10, by Cherie L. Spehar, describes the use of a different but quite creative approach—one combining standard play therapy and expressive arts interventions with therapeutic writing and mindfulness-based techniques—in confronting and overcoming adversity; the chapter includes an interesting adolescent case example and samples of both techniques and therapeutic dialogue.

We three coeditors are grateful to our chapter contributors for sharing their considerable expertise and experience with all those who work in the field of play therapy and child mental health. Our anticipated audience includes social workers, psychologists, and psychiatrists who work in a wide range of settings—schools, clinics, private practice, hospitals, foster care, and residential treatment, to name just a few.

Finally, another factor motivating us to compile this book has been the bombardment of the child mental health field in professional conferences and literature with an exclusive focus on child trauma. Although there is no denying that mental health professionals are invariably confronted with far too many trauma cases, the other side of the coin—the resilience, strength, and "islands of competence" in our children, not to mention their awe-inspiring spirit—has not, unfortunately, received the same emphasis. Practitioners sometimes come away from conference presentations that seem to focus solely on documenting and detailing trauma feeling as demoralized and hopeless as their child and family clients do. One of our respected colleagues stated that she had decided not to attend future conferences because of "feeling hammered by trauma, trauma, and trauma!" This book was conceived in the spirit of hopefulness and optimism that has sustained and inspired us as coeditors, as well as our highly seasoned and widely acclaimed contributors. Our collective aim has been to inspire and enhance hope in younger professionals—four of whom, in fact, have contributed greatly to this volume.

Contents

xiii

Play Therapy Interventions
to Enhance Resilience

Part I

INTRODUCTION

Chapter 1

The Power of Mindsets

*Guideposts for a Resilience-Based
Treatment Approach*

ROBERT BROOKS
SAM GOLDSTEIN

In this chapter, we examine two key concepts that guide our therapeutic interventions with children and adolescents: "resilience" and
"mindsets." These concepts serve as a foundation for the strength-based
approach to which we subscribe. They are not restricted to one theoretical position (e.g., psychodynamic or cognitive-behavioral); rather,
they can be applied to various therapeutic models and strategies, including the play therapy techniques that are the subject of this book (see
Seymour, Chapter 2, this volume, for specific properties of play that
promote resilience). Stuart Brown (2009), founder of the National Institute for Play, has stated in regard to imaginative play: "Throughout
life, imagination remains a key to emotional resilience and creativity"
(p. 87).

FOUR WAVES IN THE STUDY OF RESILIENCE

During the past 25 years, there has been a heightened interest in the
study of resilience in children and adolescents, and of the ways in which
this concept might be applied to both clinical and nonclinical populations (Beardslee & Podorefsky, 1988; Brooks, 2011; Brooks & Brooks,
2014; Brooks, Brooks, & Goldstein, 2012; Brooks & Goldstein, 2001,

2007, 2011; Crenshaw, 2010; Fagan, 1999; Goldstein & Brooks, 2013; Goldstein, Brooks, & DeVries, 2013; Masten, 2001; Prince-Embury & Saklofske, 2013; Werner & Smith, 2001). This interest has included taking an interactionist perspective to examine the role parents play in fostering resilience and managing risks in the lives of their children (Skinner, Pitzer, & Steele, 2013; Taylor & Conger, 2014). Concomitantly, there has also been an increased interest in identifying factors involved in the neurobiology and physiology of resilience and adaptation in children (Karatoreos & McEwen, 2013).

Wright, Masten, and Narayan (2013) have described four distinct phases or "waves" in resilience research. Initially, the emphasis was on understanding those factors within individuals who had encountered and coped successfully with significant adversity in their lives. A second wave examined developmental processes that contributed to resilience. This wave paralleled the emergence of developmental psychopathology and involved paying increased attention to contextual and developmental variables and not simply to within-person factors.

Wright and colleagues (2013) have termed the third wave "intervening to foster resilience," which encompassed both intervention and prevention approaches. These authors noted, "Using lessons from the first two waves, investigators of the third wave began to translate the basic science of resilience that was emerging into actions intended to promote resilience" (p. 27). The fourth and current wave is focused on "multilevel dynamics and the many processes linking genes, neurobiological adaptation, brain development, behavior, and context at multiple levels" (p. 30). It involves the study of resilience from many vantage points, including genes, gene–environment interaction, and social interaction.

The content of this chapter is most identifiable with the third wave, though it has obvious roots in the first two waves. However, we recognize that the fourth wave involves an exciting multidisciplinary, multilevel approach that will provide increased information about the many forces contributing to resilience in children and adolescents.

While the focus of this chapter is on therapeutic interventions, the framework we propose can also be applied within a prevention perspective. The principles we outline for nurturing a "resilient mindset" in youth in treatment can be extended to environments outside the therapy office—that is, our homes and schools—to assist all youth in managing their current and future problems more effectively.

In articulating the dimensions of our work, we strongly advocate that as an integral part of the treatment process, therapists interact closely with parents and teachers, unless there are contraindications for doing so in the particular dynamics of a situation. Close collaboration between a therapist and significant adults in a child's life affords the therapist an opportunity to articulate the tenets of a strength-based approach with these other caregivers, so that they can facilitate the development of resilience in the child.

INVULNERABLE CHILDREN?

Before we introduce the other essential concept of our work (namely, mindsets), it is important to describe a shift that has occurred in our understanding of resilience—a shift that we believe can provide encouragement and hope for therapists in their work with challenging youth.

The earliest studies of resilience examined the lives of children who had experienced significant adversity (e.g., emotional, physical, or sexual abuse; parenting by adults with emotional disorders), but now as adolescents or adults were faring well. This population was frequently given the label "invulnerable" (Anthony & Cohler, 1987), which could easily be interpreted to imply that they were "superboys" or "supergirls" who possessed unusual inborn powers that allowed them to overcome the hardships they encountered. To apply this label to a small, select group of children could lead to the incorrect conclusion that the vast majority of children (those not born with these "superpowers") would be incapable of overcoming childhood hardship and trauma.

Masten (2001), in an often-quoted article that parallels her description of the different waves of the study of resilience, eloquently challenged the notion that extraordinary powers must be involved in displaying resilience. She stated:

> Resilience does not come from rare and special qualities, but from the everyday magic of ordinary, normative human resources in the minds, brains, and bodies of children, in their families, and in their communities. . . . The conclusion that resilience emerges from ordinary processes offers a far more optimistic outlook for action than the idea that rare and extraordinary processes are involved. The task before us now is to delineate how adaptive systems develop, how they operate under diverse conditions, how they work for or against success for a given child in his or her environmental and developmental context, and how they can be protected, restored, facilitated, and nurtured in the lives of children. (p. 235)

Masten's view, to which we enthusiastically subscribe, offers a more hopeful perspective through its questioning of the assumption that only a small number of children possess certain extraordinary attributes, and that these attributes are necessary to master adversity. The shift from the notion of invulnerability to one of "ordinary magic" has far-reaching implications for clinicians as they assess the potential for resilience of each child they see in therapy.

This shift in perspective is not confined to children. Bonanno (2004) has arrived at a conclusion similar to Masten's, primarily from his study of adults who have experienced trauma and loss. He has observed:

> A review of the available literature on loss and violent or life-threatening events clearly indicates that the vast majority of individuals exposed to such events do not exhibit chronic symptom profiles and that many and, in some cases, the majority show the type of healthy functioning suggestive of the resilience trajectory. (p. 22)

In his thought-provoking book *The Other Side of Sadness*, Bonanno (2009) has offered this opinion:

> What is perhaps most intriguing about resilience is not how prevalent it is; rather it is that we are consistently surprised by it. I have to admit that sometimes even I am amazed by how resilient humans are, and I have been working with loss and trauma survivors for years. (p. 47)

Masten's and Bonanno's positions support the belief that all individuals, not just a special few, possess the capacity to become resilient. Such a belief offers, as Masten (2001) noted, a "far more optimistic outlook." It also serves as a challenge to therapists to identify and implement strategies to bring this "ordinary magic" to fruition in all youngsters.

Most, if not all, child therapists would express as an important treatment goal their patients' becoming increasingly resilient. Different clinicians and researchers may possess varying definitions of "resilience" (Goldstein & Brooks, 2013), but generally it has been understood as a child's achievement of positive developmental outcomes and avoidance of maladaptive outcomes when confronted by adverse conditions (Rutter, 2006; Wyman et al., 1999).

In an earlier publication, Brooks and Goldstein (2001) offered the following as characteristics of resilience: the capacities to deal effectively with stress and pressure; to cope with everyday challenges; to rebound from disappointments, mistakes, trauma, and adversity; to develop clear and realistic goals; to solve problems; to interact comfortably with others; and to treat oneself and others with respect and dignity.

A guiding principle in each interaction that adults have with children—whether in homes, schools, or therapists' offices—should be to strengthen these attributes, which we subsume under the concept of a "resilient mindset." This leads us to the topic of "mindsets" and its relevance for therapists.

THE POWER OF MINDSETS

The concept of "mindsets" has become a prominent topic of study, especially with the emergence of the field of "positive psychology." For example, Dweck's book, *Mindset* (2006), distinguishes between a "fixed" and a "growth" outlook. The research of Seligman and his colleagues on "learned helplessness" and "learned optimism" as well as resilience (Reivich & Shatte, 2002; Seligman, 1990, 1995) has underpinnings in attribution theory, which is basically about mindsets; attribution research examines how people understand the reasons for their successes and mistakes (Weiner, 1974).

We have noted (Brooks & Goldstein, 2001) that resilient children possess certain qualities and/or ways of viewing themselves and the world that are not apparent in youngsters who have not been successful in meeting challenges. The assumptions that children make about themselves and others influence the behaviors and skills they develop. In turn, these behaviors and skills influence the children's assumptions, so that a dynamic process is constantly operating. A child's set of assumptions may be classified as a "mindset."

Identifying the components of a resilient mindset, which are described in greater detail below, provides invaluable guidance for therapists as they initiate interventions with their child patients and/or with the significant caregivers in these children's lives. In fact, all adults who strive to develop resilience in children will benefit from such guidance. Although the outcome of a specific situation may be important, even more vital are the lessons learned from the process of dealing with each issue or problem. The knowledge gained in this process provides the basis for further enhancement of resilience and further positive development (Goldstein et al., 2013).

In discussing the concept of mindsets, it is important to appreciate that not only do we possess assumptions about ourselves, but—whether we realize it or not—we are constantly making assumptions about the behavior of others. These assumptions, even if unstated, have a significant impact in determining the quality of our relationships with children and the positive or negative climates that are created in home, school, therapeutic, and other environments. We believe that a main task of therapists is to replace negative mindsets in children and their caregivers with mindsets that nurture resilience and hope.

As therapists, we must be open to examining our own mindsets about particular youth. How do we understand the various behaviors of children? What emotions do different children evoke in us? In our workshops, we often ask, "Have parents ever called you to say that their child is ill and won't be able to come in for his/her appointment, and after you reply that you hope the child feels better, you feel a sense of relief that the appointment has been canceled?"

Many clinicians laugh when they hear this question, since most have experienced that emotion, thought, and response. We then inquire, "But why would you feel that sense of relief?" Typical answers are that a therapist is uncertain about what he/she is doing in therapy with a particular child patient, or that there has been little if any treatment progress, or that the child is very provocative and elicits anger. Whatever the reason, it is important to realize that children can sense the negative (or positive) mindsets of their therapist or other adults.

Clinical Case Example: "Punishing a Suffering Child"

The following case vignette is a vivid illustration of the impact of mindsets in determining a mother's behavior toward a child, as well as the significance of therapeutic interventions to change counterproductive childrearing mindsets and practices. Janet Norton, the single mother of 5-year-old Amanda, contacted me (Robert Brooks) and said during the initial phone call, "I'm desperate." She described how, prior to becoming a parent, she told herself that she would never resort to corporal punishment as a disciplinary tactic. Yet she was currently spanking Amanda several times a day. She asserted, "It's the only way she'll listen to me, and even that doesn't last too long."

In her first appointment, Janet described Amanda as a very challenging child to satisfy from birth—one who often had tantrums, especially when she did not get what she wanted. "Everything is a struggle with Amanda. Nothing pleases her. Things would be so much easier if only she would cooperate more with what I ask her to do. I don't think I'm asking too much of her."

In listening to Janet's description of Amanda, and guided by an appreciation of the influence that mindsets have on our reactions to different people and situations, I asked, "How do you understand Amanda's behavior or why she acts the way she does?"

Janet hesitated and then replied, "I would tell you, but I think you would think I was crazy."

"Crazy for telling me how you understand Amanda's behavior?"

"Yes."

Again, directed by the ways in which mindsets influence our behaviors, I inquired, "Do you know why I asked about how you understood Amanda's behavior?" (We often pose this kind of question to patients, as a way of both beginning a discussion about mindsets and developing a collaborative relationship in which ideas and comments are shared and understood.)

Janet thought for a moment and answered, "I'm not certain."

I responded, "In my experience, how we understand or interpret someone else's behavior—what I often refer to as our 'mindset'—will determine how we respond to that person."

"That certainly makes sense, but what I'm going to say may still seem crazy. Sometimes I feel that Amanda has a personal vendetta against me—that it's like she's always thinking of ways to upset me."

My initial response was to tell Janet that I knew it took a great deal of courage for her to share this view—the moment I used the word "courage," Janet seemed to become more relaxed—and while a "personal vendetta" might be one explanation, there might be other explanations as well. (Aware of Janet's anxiety that I would indeed experience her "personal vendetta" interpretation as a sign of her being crazy, I was careful not to judge this explanation, but rather to offer another possibility.)

Janet was eager to hear my alternative explanation, which involved a discussion of the different temperaments with which children are born. Citing the seminal work of Chess and Thomas (1987), I said that while some children are born with what researchers have labeled "easy" temperaments, others possess temperaments that are seen as "difficult." I told Janet that, according to her description, Amanda met many of the criteria for this latter label.

As the discussion continued, Janet wondered whether a child like Amanda, born with a difficult temperament, would always display this kind of temperament even into her teen and adult years. I offered realistic reassurance by noting that once adults are aware that a child has certain challenging temperamental qualities, there are techniques they can use to lessen these negative qualities.

Janet then plaintively said, "So I guess that many of the things I've spanked her about were really things she did not have control over."

"Yes, but that doesn't mean we can't help her to gain more control and be more cooperative now, without having to spank her."

Janet teared up and offered a very poignant comment: "As I think of all we've talked about, all I can think about is that I've been *punishing a suffering child*."

I empathized with Janet and added, "But that's before you really knew about temperament or different strategies to deal with children who are more difficult to parent. We can begin to consider other strategies for interacting with Amanda that do not involve spanking."

Janet was very motivated to learn these other strategies. As she did, both her confidence as a parent and her relationship with Amanda noticeably improved. She no longer spanked her daughter, observing, "Why would anyone want to spank a suffering child?"

The shift in mindset from a "personal vendetta" to a "suffering child" prompted an entirely different parental approach, which would not have been possible without this change in perspective. In turn, the shift in mindset was reinforced by the positive changes that occurred in Amanda's behavior. Janet developed a more understanding, satisfying relationship with her daughter, and Amanda responded in kind.

THE CHARACTERISTICS
OF A RESILIENT MINDSET

Given the impact of mindsets in determining our behavior, we propose that a major goal for psychotherapists is to reinforce a mindset in patients that is associated with hope and resilience. This goal will be facilitated if therapists identify the attributes of what Brooks and Goldstein (2001) have labeled a "resilient mindset" and nurture these attributes, both in the therapy setting and in consultation with significant adults in a youth's life.

A resilient mindset consists of the following noteworthy characteristics that are associated with specific skills. Resilient children:

- Feel loved and accepted.
- Have learned to set realistic goals and expectations and goals for themselves.
- Are able to define the aspects of their lives over which they have control and to focus their energy and attention on those, rather than on factors over which they have little if any influence.
- Believe that they have the ability to solve problems and make informed decisions.
- Take realistic credit for their successes and achievements, but acknowledge the input and support of adults for these successes.

- View mistakes, setbacks, and obstacles as challenges to confront and master, rather than as stressors to avoid.
- Recognize and accept their vulnerabilities and weaknesses, seeing these as areas for improvement, rather than as unchangeable flaws.
- Recognize, enjoy, and use their strengths, or what we call their "islands of competence."
- Feel comfortable with and relate well to both peers and adults.
- Believe that they make a positive difference in the lives of others.

The Importance of Serving as a Charismatic Adult

A key to being an effective therapist (or parent or teacher) is to view each interaction with a child as an opportunity to reinforce one or more of the characteristics listed above. As noted above, these characteristics serve as guideposts in our therapeutic interactions with children. We must never underestimate the impact that any of our interactions, including those in play therapy, can have on a child. A basic research finding is that resilience is rooted in the relationships that children experience with caring adults (Brooks & Goldstein, 2001, 2004). The late psychologist Julius Segal (1988), whose work focused on factors that assisted children to master adversity, eloquently noted:

> From studies conducted around the world, researchers have distilled a number of factors that enable such children of misfortune to beat the heavy odds against them. One factor turns out to be the presence in their lives of a *charismatic adult*—a person with whom they can identify and from whom they gather strength. (p. 3)

Segal's notion of a "charismatic adult" is thought-provoking. It prompts therapists to ask themselves: "At the end of each therapy session, is my patient stronger because of things I've said or done, or is my patient less strong and hopeful? Has my patient gathered strength from me?" It also highlights what many clinicians and researchers have found—namely, that resilience is rooted in children's relationships and connections with caring adults in their lives.

Clinical Case Example: The Therapist as a Charismatic Adult

The power of the relationship a child can develop with a therapist, even in the face of limited therapeutic progress, is well exemplified in the work I (Sam Goldstein) did with Steven. Steven was a bright but impulsive and extremely oppositional 9-year-old. He and his siblings had been abandoned by their parents, who had schizophrenia; the children were subsequently placed in foster care. Steven's coping strategies were such that he quickly burned out foster parents, due to his strong-willed opposition to even the most minor requests, combined with his verbal precocity and ability to quickly frustrate even the most well-meaning adult. On his first visit to see me, Steven was sitting in the waiting room reading a book. I soon learned that reading was a powerful protective factor for Steven: He could withdraw into his book when the stresses around him became excessive. I invited Steven to come into my office, to which Steven responded, "Sure, when I finish this book."

Steven was about halfway through what appeared to be a very large novel in the Harry Potter series. Rather than confront Steven, I said, "Well, that's fine. I have some reading to do also. Do you mind if I pull up a chair and sit here and read with you until you are ready to come in?"

This comment took Steven by surprise (an unexpected reply often draws reflection and attention). Steven responded affirmatively. Steven kept glancing at me as I read a magazine. After a few minutes, Steven closed the book and exclaimed, "This isn't a very interesting book. Let's go into your office."

Steven proceeded over the first few visits to test me repeatedly by sitting in my chair, opening my drawers, and asking questions about my personal life. I responded patiently to all of these questions and actions. Basic rules were set that Steven agreed to and followed during weekly therapy visits. Even after multiple visits, however, when I would ask questions about Steven's week or activities, Steven would reply, "That's private." Nearly everything I sought to talk about or discuss, Steven considered "private."

Yet Steven quickly became attached to me, even though he would not talk or participate very much in therapeutic play. His foster mother reported that he never forgot a visit, often reminding her the night before. When I had to miss a week after approximately 8–10 visits due to travel, Steven immediately complained that this was *his* time and he wanted to be seen. Eventually Steven's attachment to my adhering to our schedule progressed to willingness to share his thoughts and feelings. This willingness also resulted in an improvement in Steven's behavior. I had evidently become a charismatic adult in Steven's life.

Strategies for Encouraging Parents and Teachers to Become Charismatic Adults

Therapists, in explaining the notion of a "charismatic adult" to children's parents and/or teachers, can ask these caregivers to consider similar questions:

"When I put my children to bed at night, do I ask, 'Are my children stronger because of things I've said or done today, or are they less strong? Have they gathered strength from me?' "

"At the end of the school day, do I as a teacher ask, 'Are all of the students in my classroom stronger because of things I've said or done today, or are they less strong? Have they gathered strength from me?' "

These are not easy questions to answer, especially since the concept and measurement of "strength" are far from precise. However, when parents, educators, and therapists consider whether they are serving as charismatic adults, such consideration elicits this basic question: "What do I say or do to serve in that role?"

One answer resides in identifying and applying those strategies that reinforce the attributes of a resilient mindset. We believe that a commonality among therapists, even those holding different theoretical positions, can be found in an understanding and reinforcement of the characteristics of a resilient mindset in their patients. For example, Crenshaw and his colleagues have demonstrated that the use of play therapy represents one therapeutic approach with children that can be used to reinforce resilience in the face of hardship and trauma (Crenshaw, 2008, 2010; Malchiodi & Crenshaw, 2014).

GUIDEPOSTS FOR NURTURING A RESILIENT MINDSET

We have selected several of the main attributes of a resilient mindset as guideposts for therapists to follow as they strive to have their patients gather strength from them.

Encouraging the Belief That Adults Can Be Supportive and Helpful

The relationships therapists develop with children are of paramount importance in helping the children feel safe, secure, accepted, and loved—prerequisites for the emergence of resilience. This statement may appear so obvious that some may question the necessity for its inclusion here. However, our purpose in emphasizing this point is to promote consideration of the different actions therapists can initiate to help children feel safe and accepted in their offices. If children do not perceive adults as caring and supportive—if they sense that adults can be harmful and judgmental—it will be difficult for them to accept adults into their lives, and thereby will rob them of an opportunity to become resilient.

A major skill for therapists and other adults to demonstrate if they are to foster positive feelings in children toward their caregivers is to demonstrate empathy. That is, the adults should always attempt to see the world through the children's eyes. In our clinical practices and workshops, we invite therapists, parents, and educators to reflect upon particular questions to help bring focus to the concept of empathy:

"How would I feel if someone said or did to me what I just said or did to my patient [child, student]?"

"When I say or do things with my patients [children, students], do I communicate in a way that will help them realize I care about them, so that they will be more receptive to listening to me?"

"How would I hope my patients [children, students] describe me?"

"What have I done on a regular basis so that my patients [children, students] are likely to describe me in the ways I hope they would?" (This particular question encourages adults to consider specific plans of action to enrich their relationships with children they are raising or with whom they are working.)

"How would my patients [children, students] actually describe me, and how close is that to how I hope they would describe me?"

"If there is a discrepancy between the hoped-for and actual descriptions, what steps must I take to lessen that discrepancy?" (Another question to prompt a plan of action.)

Clinical Case Example: Facilitating Parental Empathy

An example of how these questions were used to help parents become more empathic and charismatic adults in the life of their child took place with Sally, a shy 8-year-old. Sally was frequently reminded by her parents, Sue and Alan, to say hello to people. The first question that greeted Sally after school was "Did you speak with anyone in school today? If you don't make the effort, you're not going to have any friends." These kinds of comments backfired, prompting Sally to become increasingly anxious.

Sue and Alan were understandably worried about Sally and desired her to be more outgoing. However, they failed to appreciate that Sally's cautious demeanor was an inborn temperamental trait that could not be overcome by exhorting her to say hello to others or make friends. Each reminder on their part intensified Sally's discomfort; increased her feeling that she had disappointed her parents; and compromised the development of a warm, supportive relationship between Sally and her parents.

Parent counseling focused on changing Sue and Alan's mindset about Sally, so that she would experience her parents as supportive rather than critical. They were asked to consider the impact their current actions and words were having on their daughter. If they were shy, how would they feel if someone said to them, "You have to make an effort to speak with other people, or you won't have friends and you'll be lonely"? Reflecting on these questions at first startled Sue and Alan, but then served as a catalyst to help them develop a more empathic stance toward their daughter.

The parents asked how they might approach Sally and whether they should avoid saying anything at all about her shy behavior. They were encouraged not to avoid the subject, but rather to help Sally by express- ing empathy and by having her feel they were on her side rather than judging her. In parent counseling, they learned to inform Sally that they knew it was not easy for her to say hello to people she didn't know; they also began to add that it was not easy for other children as well. Such statements, expressed in a genuine fashion, conveyed empathy and also helped to normalize the problem Sally was facing. Normalizing a prob- lem permits children as well as adults to feel that they are not alone—a very reassuring feeling.

Sue and Alan then created a problem-solving atmosphere, which (as we highlight below) is a major facilitator of resilience. They suggested to Sally that perhaps the three of them working together could figure out small steps that she could begin taking to make it less difficult for her to greet others. They also offered realistic hope by asserting, "Many kids who have trouble saying hello when they're young find it easier as they get older."

These changes contributed to a more positive relationship between Sally and her parents, and encouraged Sally to take the "small steps" Sue and Alan began to suggest. Sally's perception that her parents were supportive rather than judgmental was a significant shift in her mindset, and it allowed her to venture forth more confidently in her daily interac- tions with others.

Strategies for Enhancing Empathy

In conducting therapy, clinicians can offer comments that represent their wish to be empathic and to understand the perspective of their patients. Comments such as the following, timed for the appropriate moments, frequently lessen defensiveness and enrich the therapist– patient alliance:

> "If you ever feel I'm not understanding something you're trying to tell me, please let me know."
> "If you ever feel I'm being critical of you or judging you, please let me know since that would never be my intention." (We have found

this comment to be very powerful with children, as well as their
parents, who are often poised to feel that they are being judged.)
"If I ever ask you a question and you're not certain why, don't hesitate to ask me why I'm asking the question." (A similar statement was used in the earlier example with Janet Norton, to
inquire about her understanding of her daughter's behavior.)

These and similar statements should not be seen as rigid scripts to be
produced indiscriminately, but rather as a sincere reflection of a therapist's wish to develop a warm, caring, and empathic relationship with
children and their families.

In addition, as Brooks and Brooks (Chapter 3, this volume) describe,
many empathic communications with children can be expressed very
effectively via play, storytelling, and metaphors (Brooks, 1981, 1985).

Before we leave the theme of the therapist–patient relationship, it
is important to consider the possible obstacles to being more empathic
and nurturing in this relationship. Therapists must recognize that it is
usually easier to be empathic and caring toward patients who are cooperative and eager to enter into a warm relationship. As we have often
noted in our writings and workshops, a far greater challenge is to be
empathic and to reach out to individuals with whom therapists are upset
or disappointed, or who push them away when they attempt to be helpful. To gain their trust will require acceptance and time; trust cannot be
acquired overnight.

Encouraging the Belief That We Have More Control over Our Reactions to Events Than We May Realize

Developing an outlook of "personal control" in children is an essential
feature of helping them develop resilience. In identifying personal control as a key ingredient of a resilient mindset, we (Brooks & Goldstein,
2004) offered the following description of this concept:

> Taking ownership of our behavior and becoming more resilient
> requires us to recognize that we are the authors of our lives. We must
> not seek our happiness by asking someone else to change, but instead
> always ask, *What is it that I can do differently to change the situa-
> tion?* Assuming personal control and responsibility is a fundamental
> underpinning of a resilient mindset, one that affects all other features
> of this mindset. (p. 7)

Although this statement focuses primarily on resilience in adults, it is
equally relevant for our interventions with children. As therapists, we

should be sensitive to assessing whether children and/or their families are burdened by a victim's mentality. Such a mentality is dominated by thoughts and feelings associated with a sense of helplessness and hopelessness. Or do they entertain the notion that while negative events over which they have little if any control have transpired in their lives, what they do have control over is their attitude toward and reaction to these events?

Clinical Case Examples: Facilitating Personal Control

Sean, a 9-year-old boy with a diagnosis of attention-deficit/hyperactivity disorder (ADHD), was struggling not only in school, but with the recent divorce of his parents. In one session, frustrated and angry, he asked, "Why did God choose me to be the one with ADHD?"

It is not unusual for children or adults faced with adversity to ask, "Why me?" or "Why my child?" The problem is exacerbated when the "Why?" question continues to dominate their thinking year after year. Eventually, feelings of helplessness and victimization may become the prominent features of these persons' mindsets. Gerber, Ginsberg, and Reiff (1992) studied adults with learning disabilities and found that those who were more successful in different arenas of their lives had adopted this outlook: "I had no control over being born with learning problems, but I do have control in terms of how effectively I cope with those problems." The less successful adults kept moaning, "Why did I have to be born with learning disabilities?"

So how might a therapist respond to Sean's question, "Why did God choose me to be the one with ADHD?" When asked what he thought, Sean could offer no explanation. Gerber and colleagues' (1992) findings offer direction. Sean's therapist offered the following resilience-based response: "We're not sure why some kids have ADHD and some don't, but the encouraging news is that now that we know you have ADHD, there are things that can be done to help kids like yourself and others with ADHD to be more successful."

It is important for a therapist to understand both a child's and a parent's notion of personal control. This understanding may be facilitated by using a particular mindset model that we have mentioned earlier in this chapter—namely, attribution theory (Weiner, 1974). Children who struggle with self-esteem and are not very hopeful or resilient tend to believe that any success that comes their way is based on luck, chance, or fate. They tend to attribute success to factors outside their control, which lessens the probability of future accomplishment. In contrast, youngsters with a more positive outlook will give the adults in their lives credit for their assistance, but they basically believe—and not in a narcissistic way—that their success is predicated in great part on their own effort and resources.

In terms of setbacks and mistakes, children with low self-esteem are prone to attribute mistakes to things they cannot change (e.g., low intelligence), prompting feelings of hopelessness and the emergence of self-defeating coping strategies (e.g., quitting at difficult points, not even attempting certain challenges, blaming others). Children who are secure attribute mistakes to situations from which they can learn rather than feel defeated. They are more likely to use mistakes to establish realistic goals and strategies for success.

An understanding of a child's beliefs about personal control can begin during the assessment phase. Samantha, a 12-year-old girl, was referred to me (Robert Brooks) because of her feelings of sadness and loneliness, coupled with low self-esteem and learning problems in school. During the first interview, she immediately described her distress and obvious sense of hopelessness and helplessness: "I'm not very popular, I have trouble in school, and I'm terrible at sports. That's why I stay in my room a lot."

In response to my questions, Samantha acknowledged that she wished things were different. I asked her what she would like to change.

Samantha readily responded, "I wish I was as pretty as the other girls, and that I was popular and could play sports and get good grades in school."

As the discussion continued, I wondered if there was ever a time that Samantha felt more successful. Her reply could have been taken directly from a book illustrating the tenets of attribution theory. Samantha talked about a time when another girl complimented her, but she dismissed this gesture by contending, "She felt sorry for me." She also minimized a good grade she received on an English paper with the comment, "I think the teacher felt sorry for me."

Therapy with Samantha focused on changing these self-defeating attributions or assumptions. As I frequently do with children and adolescents, I explained—in language that Samantha could understand—the concept of mindsets and their impact on her behavior. A therapeutic goal was to modify Samantha's mindset by incorporating a more hopeful outlook. As this goal was being realized, Samantha attempted new scripts (Brooks & Goldstein, 2001, 2004) that led to positive outcomes. She "rehearsed" in therapy, including through the use of dolls and play, different ways of approaching a couple of girls with interests similar to her own. She also received assistance from a tutor, especially about preparing for tests, which led to improved grades. In place of sports, she cultivated an interest in painting and enrolled in an art class in a museum.

With each positive result, I was very active in asking, "Why do you think that what you did was successful?" Samantha understood why I was asking, and soon she would say playfully, "I know what you're going to ask me."

"You do?"

"You were going to ask why I thought I was successful?"

With humor I replied, "Wow! I must be really predictable. But let me ask anyway: Why do you think you were successful?"

This dialogue not only demonstrates the use of humor in therapy with a child, but illustrates that an important shift in Samantha's outlook occurred when she could acknowledge that her success was based not only on the help of others, but—just as importantly, if not more so—on her own effort.

Strategies for Reinforcing Personal Control

Therapists can offer suggestions to parents and teachers for how best to reinforce personal control in children. For instance, these adults can call attention to a child's efforts in determining the outcome of an event. The following are but a few examples of such feedback:

> "You really put in a lot of time and effort to learn those spelling words, and it showed on how nicely you did on this test."
> "I know it wasn't easy for you to memorize the lines for the school play, but all the hours you spent memorizing your part really paid off."
> "Do you remember that the last time we went to the restaurant, it wasn't easy for you to wait for the meal, and you started to yell? We spoke with you about it, and this time you waited so nicely. We appreciate how you behaved."

Since we believe that, whenever possible, parents and teachers should be active participants in the treatment program, therapists should also be sensitive to reinforcing personal control within these caregivers. As children show progress, therapists must give genuine credit to the role that parents and teachers have played. Simple comments such as "Your changing your discipline approach has certainly led to a change in Jack's behavior," or "Your allowing Maria to read to younger students has really led to a boost in her self-esteem and motivation," spotlight the significant role of the adult in modifying the child's behavior.

Encouraging the Belief That Problems Can Be Solved Instead of Becoming Overwhelming

Intimately tied to the task of reinforcing a belief in personal control, but deserving special attention, are the acquisition and use of problem-solving skills. If children act before they think, and if they don't consider the consequences of their behavior, they will have difficulty developing effective coping strategies and a sense of personal control. Many of our patients demonstrate difficulties with problem solving, and as a result feel lost and confused. In contrast, resilient youngsters are able to identify problems, consider different solutions, select what they believe will be the most effective solution, and learn from the outcome (Shure, 1996; Shure & Aberson, 2013).

Shure (1996), one of the foremost experts on reinforcing problem-solving abilities in children, has found that even preschool children can be assisted to develop and apply these skills. Shure and other professionals believe that well-intentioned adults often rush in too quickly to tell children what to do, rather than enlisting their input when the children are faced with challenges. When children are afforded an opportunity to initiate their own plans of action with the guidance of adults, their feelings of ownership and personal control are reinforced.

Clinical Case Example: Facilitating Problem Solving

The ability to solve problems at a young age was developed with 6-year-old Carl, a boy diagnosed with ADHD. In his attempts to make friends, he often invaded the space of his peers by giving them hugs—an action that, not surprisingly, usually backfired.

I (Robert Brooks) asked Carl whether he thought that his behavior was a problem. (This is a question that should always be posed, since if children or adolescents do not perceive certain behaviors as problems, then they will not be motivated to change; if a child denies that a problem really is a problem, the therapist can engage in a discussion about why the behavior in question might be problematic.) When asked this question, Carl looked sad and replied, "Big problem. I might not have any friends. But I just forget, and I hug kids."

When asked if he could think of a way to begin to solve the problem, Carl did not hesitate to say, "I need reminders."

I inquired, "What do you mean by 'reminders'?"

Carl said, "I think if the teacher reminded me each morning not to hug another kid, it would help me to remember."

"That's a great idea."

With the permission of Carl's parents, I arranged a meeting with Carl and Carl's teacher. The teacher, in an empathic and supportive way, began the meeting by telling Carl she was very pleased that he could tell me what he thought would be helpful. This comment immediately put Carl at ease.

To reinforce his problem-solving skills, the teacher then asked, "How would you like to be reminded?"

Carl said that he noticed that sometimes the teacher would touch children on their shoulders, and he thought if she did the same to him at the beginning of the day, it would be a good reminder.

She complimented him on this suggestion and then inquired, "How often would you like me to remind you?"

Carl's response was what the teacher later referred to as "precious." He was just learning to tell time, and he jumped off his chair and held one hand up and said, "When the big hand is up and when it is down," which was accompanied by his moving his hand from an up to a down position.

The decision was thus made to start this intervention the next day with reminders given every 30 minutes. At the end of the following day, Carl's mother called me to provide feedback. She said, "Carl came home very excited and said he thought the reminders were really going to work, but then he added that he thought he needed the reminders every 10 minutes."

Carl's teacher followed this suggestion. Within a few weeks, the reminders that were offered every 10 minutes were spaced back out to every 30 minutes, and then to every hour. Finally, the reminders were not needed at all. It was Carl's input that led to this problem-solving strategy—a strategy that proved very successful.

Strategies for Facilitating Problem Solving

We are often asked, "What if a child or adolescent patient is not able to say what might be helpful, or has difficulty thinking of different solutions to problems?" It is not unusual for this to occur. When it does, we suggest that a therapist respond first by saying, "Let's try to figure this out together." By asking certain questions, the therapist can then engage the child in a dialogue that will eventually produce solutions.

As Shure (1996) has advocated, parents can nurture their children's problem-solving abilities from an early age by first providing simple choices (e.g., "Do you want to wear the blue dress or the green dress?", "Do you want to take a bath first or memorize your spelling words first?"), and then moving to more complex choices and decisions.

Countless situations arise in which children's input can be encouraged. The same can be done in schools, such as by inviting children to attend part or all of a parent–teacher–student conference, or by having them select what two of three homework questions to answer that they believe will help them to learn best.

Shure and Aberson (2013) have quoted the words of a parent who discovered the benefits of applying their problem-solving program: "'I learned that I as a parent can be part of the solution for my child rather than adding to the problem. Before using this approach I was trying to take power and felt powerless. Now we solve problems together'" (p. 500). In this example, both parent and child had become more resilient.

Encouraging the Belief That We All Have Strengths Even When Struggling with Problems

Resilient children do not minimize or deny problems that they have. Denial runs counter to mastery. However, in addition to acknowledging and confronting problems, youngsters who are resilient are able to identify and use their strengths, or what Brooks has called their "islands of competence" (see, e.g., Brooks & Goldstein, 2001). This metaphor represents a symbol of hope and resilience; it reminds us that all children have strengths.

We regularly ask our child and adolescent patients what they judge to be their strengths or islands of competence. If they are not certain, we reply, "That's OK. It can take time to figure out what we're good at—but it's important to figure this out." We always ask the parents and teachers of our young patients to identify the patients' strengths and discuss ways to reinforce these strengths. It is also important to ask parents what they see as their own strengths, including in the parental role. We must move from a so-called "deficit model," in which the focus is on fixing problems, to paying more than lip service to the strengths that reside in all children and adults.

Clinical Case Example: Reinforcing Strengths

I (Robert Brooks) saw 10-year-old Madison, a shy fourth grader with very low self-esteem who was often teased by other girls. Madison's mother, Abby, commented, "Sometimes I wish that Madison would stand up for herself. She always seems to live in the background." When I asked Abby what she saw as Madison's strengths, she responded quickly, "She has a beautiful singing voice. I wish she would try out for a school play."

In a meeting with Madison, I asked her what activities she enjoyed doing and what she thought she did rather well. Madison quickly answered that she didn't know, but after further discussion, she said that her mom had told her she had a nice voice. She added that when her class was singing a group song, her teacher told her afterward that she couldn't help noticing what a "strong singing voice" Madison had. I asked Madison if she would sing a song during one of our sessions. She replied that she would feel more comfortable singing and recording it at home and bringing in a copy. She did so, and I told her how impressed I was while listening to her.

This led me to encourage Madison to audition for a school play. Madison took this encouragement a step further and auditioned for a musical being sponsored by a community group that Abby had located. Madison was awarded the part she coveted, and she invited me to attend one of the performances, which I did. Madison appeared completely confident as she sang, and this experience proved to be a significant turning point in her life.

The power of the therapeutic relationship in serving as a foundation for the positive changes in Madison's life was captured years later when she contacted me after reading an article in which I was quoted in a local newspaper. She said that she had been intending to get in touch with me for a while to let me know how she was doing. She reported that she was happy in both her career and her marriage, and loved her role as a mother of two children, 6 and 8 years of age. She reminisced about her sessions with me and said, "I will never forget that you came to hear me sing. You really encouraged me to find and use my strengths."

If children are to be resilient, not only must they perceive that they have strengths; just as importantly, they must believe that their strengths are appreciated and supported by the significant adults in their lives, including their parents and teachers.

Encouraging the Belief That We Make a Positive Difference in the World

When I (Robert Brooks) was collecting material for the book *The Self-Esteem Teacher* (Brooks, 1991), I requested approximately 1,500 adults to complete an anonymous questionnaire. The first question asked them to report on a positive memory of school when they were students—something an educator said or did that boosted their self-esteem. I had not anticipated the content of the most commonly reported positive memory: being asked to help out in some fashion. The following are a few examples:

"I remember when a teacher asked me to pass out the milk and straws."

"I felt so good when a teacher asked me to tutor a younger child."

"I remember when a teacher told me I was a good artist and asked me to draw some signs as part of an anti-litter campaign."

Clinical Case Example: Helping Youth to Help Others

When concluding psychotherapy with a child, I (Sam Goldstein) appeal to the child for help during the closing visit. I explain that there will be other children coming to see me who may have similar problems, and that the support from someone who is now feeling, doing, and behaving better will be very important to children who are first entering therapy. I then ask the child to consider drawing a picture, writing a note, or making a poster that can be given to another child. Below is a poem written by 16-year-old Devin, expressing his feelings about living with autism. He wrote this for me after completing a course of supportive psychotherapy:

Were They but There at Night

There is a boulder field where every stone
Is a glazed, glittering gem, like stars fallen from the sky.
All except one, a plain grey rock alone in the center
Feeling excluded and shunned.
People come, tourists, painters, photographers, collectors
To view each shining boulder, a pleasure to the beholder.
Ooh! Ahh! Look at this one! Come quick!
Pockets bulge with fragments and paint cans run dry.
But the grey rock remains ignored
An ugly blotch on a sweeping mural.
The sun sets, everyone leaves,
And they miss the centerpiece of the field.
For when night falls, the grey rock in the center
It glows in the dark.

(Reprinted by permission of Devin Teichert.)

Strategies for Helping Youth to Help Others

Brooks and Goldstein (2001, 2004) have proposed that there is an inborn need to help that continues to be a powerful force throughout the lifespan. As Werner (1993) captured in her longitudinal research, resilience was nurtured when children were provided opportunities to help others, or "contributory activities" (Brooks & Goldstein, 2001). Involvement in these activities nurtures a very important belief in a child, one that reinforces a sense of purpose: namely, "What I am doing adds to the well-being and happiness of others."

We observe that too often adults preach to children about being more caring and compassionate. There should be less lecturing about these admirable qualities and more opportunities to display them. Situations occur that allow therapists to emphasize "contributory activities." For example, when children arrive at impressive strategies for solving particular problems, a therapist can call attention to the effectiveness of the strategy. We have said to our child patients, "That's such a good idea, I'd love to use it with other kids. I think it will really be helpful to them."

We are frequently asked by parents at our workshops what they can do to develop compassion and responsibility in their children. One response we offer is to ask parents to consider how their children would reply to the following questions:

"What are the ways you have seen your parents help other people in the past few months?"
"What activities have you been involved with together with your parents in the past few months in which you have helped other people?"

Children are more likely to become altruistic and caring if they not only observe their parents helping others, but are enlisted in such roles themselves. We advise parents to say when they are attempting to involve their children, "We need your help," rather than "Remember to do your chores." Not surprisingly, most children do not like to do "chores," but are especially willing to engage in the same activities when they are cast in terms of helping others. Parents who encourage their children's participation in charitable endeavors, such as walks to end hunger or to support research on AIDS or breast cancer, are supporting a resilient mindset.

In our consultations with parents and teachers, we have emphasized that charitable activities can be used to reinforce other components of a resilient mindset, such as problem solving (e.g., deciding what charity to support and how to raise money for the charity), empathy (e.g., taking the perspective of the people being assisted), and applying one's "islands of competence" (e.g., Madison's singing in a play).

Encouraging the Belief That Mistakes Are Not Only Expectable but Also Acceptable

As we have noted earlier in our discussion of attribution theory, resilient children, though they are not thrilled when they make mistakes, view setbacks as opportunities for learning. For example, resilient children who fail a test will ask for help and/or problem-solve about more effective ways of studying. In sports, resilient children will take extra batting or fielding practice to improve their skills. These youngsters attribute mistakes to variables they can correct.

The picture is very different for children who are not resilient. They attribute mistakes to factors that they cannot change, whether they perceive these as their intelligence or an inborn lack of skills. They believe that regardless of what they do, nothing will ever change. Eventually, not wishing to face additional failure and its accompanying sense of humiliation, they often adopt self-defeating ways of coping. A boy in therapy revealed, "I'd rather hit another kid and be sent to the principal's office than have to be in the classroom where I feel like a dummy."

Clinical Case Example: Facilitating Acceptance of Mistakes

The powerful negative mindset children develop about mistakes was very well illustrated in my (Sam Goldstein's) work with Jeremy, a very bright, impulsive, inattentive 6-year-old in first grade. During the course of a clinical interview, Jeremy told me, "Teachers don't like when children make mistakes."

I inquired, "Why not?"

Jeremy responded, "They put red marks all over your paper, and what's even worse, they tell your mother."

I attempted to engage Jeremy in a discussion about the benefits of making mistakes, but Jeremy was adamant that mistakes were "bad." Helping Jeremy to begin accepting mistakes and learning from them therefore became a focus of his therapy.

Strategies for Facilitating Acceptance of/Learning from Mistakes

Therapists are in an excellent position to reinforce a positive attitude toward mistakes and lessen self-defeating behaviors in children and adolescents. They can assess children's mindsets and attributions about mistakes through direct questions or via play activities. Therapists can inquire of children the reasons they thought they were not successful at a task, what they might do differently next time (this, of course, also engages a child's problem-solving skills), and who might be available to help.

A favorite technique in our therapy or consultation activities occurs when we have helped to develop a plan of action with our child patients and/or their parents and/or their teachers. Given a particular situation, we might say, "This plan sounds great, but what if it doesn't work?" Some might wonder whether posing such a question represents a self-fulfilling prophecy for failure. It might if we did not immediately add, "What is your backup plan if it doesn't work?"

The addition of a question about a backup plan was prompted by the reactions of some of our patients or those with whom we were consulting when a plan of action proved unsuccessful. Many became frustrated and angry. It was not unusual for us to hear from teachers or parents, "We went out of our way to change things, but the child is still not willing to change"—or, as one parent lamented, "I guess this works for most parents, but I must really be doing something wrong." We learned that if people (children, parents, or teachers) are to develop a more positive attitude about mistakes, which is an essential characteristic of resilience, we must build in the possibility that failure may occur—accompanied by the message that if one strategy is unsuccessful, they can learn from that setback and then initiate other strategies.

In our consultations with teachers, we encourage them to share with their students some of their own anxieties and experiences about making mistakes when they were students. They might even discuss a time when they were embarrassed or humiliated by something one of their teachers said (students love to hear these accounts). They can then turn the discussion into a problem-solving exercise by asking, "What can I do as your teacher, and what can you do as a class, so that no one will ever feel humiliated in this class and no one will be afraid to make mistakes?"

Teachers have reported very positive results of using this exercise. One teacher informed us, "After I openly discussed the issues of mistakes and humiliation, it was the most discipline-free year I've ever had." She discovered that when children are not afraid about making mistakes, they are less likely to engage in negative behaviors in the classroom.

Parents are in an excellent position to help children from a very early age develop the belief that they can learn from mistakes. If children can incorporate this attribution for mistakes, they will become more resilient and better equipped to face challenges. To assist parents with the goal of helping their children to be less fearful of making mistakes, we ask them to consider what their children's answers would be to the following two questions:

"When your parents make a mistake, or when something doesn't go right, what do they do?"
"When you make a mistake, how do your parents respond?"

The rationale for the first question is that parents serve as significant models for handling mistakes. It is easier for children to learn to deal more effectively with setbacks if they see their parents doing so. It is very reassuring to children when they observe their parents model a problem-solving attitude toward mistakes, communicating the message through their words and actions, "What can I learn from this mistake? What can I do differently next time to be successful?"

The second question invites parents to consider whether their responses to their children's mistakes generate a healthy attitude toward mistakes or lead to greater insecurity and ineffective ways of coping. Asking children to consider other options or strategies when faced with a setback is far more effective than expressing such judgmental comments as "I told you it wouldn't work!" or "You really have to begin using your brains!"

CONCLUDING COMMENTS

We believe that one of our most important roles as therapists is that of charismatic adults. Our assumption of this role will be facilitated if we identify and reinforce the characteristics of a resilient mindset in our patients, allowing them to lead more hopeful, responsible lives. Though our formal relationship with our therapy clients may come to an end, we should always recognize that the emotional and psychological ties we create with our patients may last all their lives. Both of us routinely receive correspondence from former patients. I (Sam Goldstein) recently received an email from a young woman I worked with during her teenage years. At the time, she was struggling with depression as well as complex medical problems. She was on the verge of dropping out of school and began to engage in a variety of self-destructive behaviors. More than 20 years later, she emailed me to say that she came across my website while looking for some articles for some of her patients. She had eventually returned to school, stabilized her life, obtained a medical degree, married, and had a family of her own; she was now a pediatrician. She thanked me for my confidence in her, and remembered that I had told her she could gather the strength to be happy and make good choices.

In a note to me, another youth wrote during his young adult years: "You've always been kind and considerate of me. I appreciate your work and efforts on my behalf. I am proud to say that I am still doing very well, thanks to people like you."

One of my (Robert Brooks's) patients, Julie, whom I had not seen in 25 years, attended an evening presentation I was giving for parents in a suburb of Boston. When I saw Julie as a 10-year-old girl, she was very anxious, socially shy, and insecure. During 2 years of therapy, Julie demonstrated impressive progress, becoming increasingly self-assured and resilient. Julie and I kept in touch on a periodic basis for a few years, and I knew that she was doing very well. When she came up after my presentation, she informed me that she was happily married, had two children, and had a high-level position in the world of business. Julie then added, "I meant to write you long before tonight, but when I saw that you were speaking here, I thought it would be the perfect time to come up and thank you." She paused and with much emotion said, "I'm not certain you ever knew how important my therapy sessions with you were. I felt so accepted by you, and I will always remember the confidence you showed in me and your encouragement to face rather than run away from challenges."

Interestingly, several weeks later when I was speaking in a neighboring town, a man approached me and said, "My wife told me I just had to come and hear you—that you meant so much to her years ago." It was Julie's husband, who in his brief conversation with me appeared very warm and caring.

And I will never forget the time when one of my former child patients, now a mental health professional, gave me two books he had recently written—one in which he thanked me in the Acknowledgments, and the other in which he wrote a truly beautiful inscription that ended with these words: "You help so many find permission to learn from what is hard for them. I have tried to write this book in that spirit." What a succinct description of how therapists, in their role as charismatic adults, nurture resilient mindsets in their child patients and help them go down more hopeful, accomplished paths in life!

As therapists, we can also engage children's parents, teachers, and other caregivers to become charismatic adults. When all caregivers work in concert to nurture a resilient mindset in children, the children will be better prepared to overcome current difficulties and face new challenges with greater courage, improved skills, and enhanced perseverance.

REFERENCES

Anthony, E. J., & Cohler. B. J. (Eds.). (1987). *The invulnerable child*. New York: Guilford Press.

Beardslee, W. R., & Podorefsky, D. (1988). Resilient adolescents whose parents have serious affective and other psychiatric disorders: Importance of self-understanding and relationships. *American Journal of Psychiatry, 145,* 63–69.

Bonanno, G. A. (2004). Loss, trauma, and human resilience: Have we underestimated the human capacity to thrive after extremely aversive events? *American Psychologist, 59,* 20–28.

Bonanno, G. A. (2009). *The other side of sadness*. New York: Basic Books.

Brooks, R. (1981). Creative Characters: A technique in child therapy. *Psychotherapy, 18,* 131–139.

Brooks, R. (1985). The beginning sessions of therapy: Of messages and metaphors. *Psychotherapy, 22,* 761–769.

Brooks, R. (1991). *The self-esteem teacher*. Loveland, OH: Treehaus Communications.

Brooks, R. (2011). Building resilience by shaping mindsets. In S. Goldstein, J. Naglieri, & M. DeVries (Eds.), *Learning and attention disorders in adolescence and adulthood: Assessment and treatment* (pp. 367–404). Hoboken, NJ: Wiley.

Brooks, R., & Brooks, S. (2014). Creating resilient mindsets in children and adolescents: A strength-based approach for clinical and nonclinical populations. In S. Prince-Embury & D. H. Saklofske (Eds.), *Resilience interventions for youth in diverse populations* (pp. 59–82). New York: Springer.

Brooks, R., Brooks, S., & Goldstein, S. (2012). The power of mindsets: Nurturing engagement, motivation, and resilience in students. In S. Christenson, A. L. Resschly, & C. Wylie (Eds.), *Handbook of research on student engagement* (pp. 541–562). New York: Springer.

Brooks, R., & Goldstein, S. (2001). *Raising resilient children*. New York: McGraw-Hill.

Brooks, R., & Goldstein, S. (2004). *The power of resilience*. New York: McGraw-Hill.

Brooks, R., & Goldstein, S. (2007). *Raising a self-disciplined child*. New York: McGraw-Hill.

Brooks, R., & Goldstein, S. (2011). The power of mindsets: Raising resilient children. In G. Koocher & A. La Greca (Eds.), *The parents' guide to psychological first aid: Helping children and adolescents cope with predictable life crises* (pp. 142–150). New York: Oxford University Press.

Brown, S. (2009). *Play: How it shapes the brain, opens the imagination, and invigorates the soul*. New York: Avery.

Chess, S., & Thomas, A. (1996). *Know your child*. New York: Basic Books.

Crenshaw, D. A. (Ed.). (2008). *Child and adolescent psychotherapy: Wounded spirits and healing paths* (2nd ed.). Lanham, MD: Jason Aronson.

Crenshaw, D. A. (Ed.). (2010). *Reverence in healing: Honoring strengths without trivializing suffering*. Lanham, MD: Jason Aronson.

Dweck, C. S. (2006). *Mindset: The new psychology of success*. New York: Random House.

Fagan, D. B. (1999). Caregiving and developmental factors differentiating young at-risk urban children showing resilient versus stress-affected outcomes: A replication and extension. *Child Development, 709,* 645–659.

Gerber, P. J., Ginsberg, R., & Reiff, H. B. (1992). Identifying alterable patterns in employment success for highly successful adults with learning disabilities. *Journal of Learning Disabilities, 25,* 475–487.

Goldstein, S., & Brooks, R. (2007). *Understanding and managing children's classroom behavior: Creating resilient, sustainable classrooms* (2nd ed.). Hoboken, NJ: Wiley.

Goldstein, S., & Brooks, R. (Eds.). (2013). *Handbook of resilience in children* (2nd ed.). New York: Springer.

Goldstein, S., Brooks, R., & DeVries, M. (2013). Translating resilience theory for application with children and adolescents by parents, teachers, and mental health professionals. In S. Prince-Embury & D. H. Saklofske (Eds.), *Resilience in children, adolescents, and adults: Translating research into practice* (pp. 73–90). New York: Springer.

Karatoreos, I. N., & McEwen, B. S. (2013). Annual research review: The neurobiology and physiology of resilience and adaptation across the life course. *Journal of Child Psychology and Psychiatry, 54,* 337–347.

Malchiodi, C. A., & Crenshaw, D. A. (Eds.). (2014). *Creative arts and play therapy for attachment problems.* New York: Guilford Press.

Masten, A. S. (2001). Ordinary magic: Resilience processes in development. *American Psychologist, 56,* 227–238.

Prince-Embury, S., & Saklofske, D. H. (Eds.). (2013). *Resilience in children, adolescents, and adults: Translating research into practice.* New York: Springer.

Reivich, K., & Shatte, A. (2002). *The resilience factor.* New York: Broadway Books.

Rutter, M. (2006). Implications of resilience concepts for scientific understanding. *Annals of the New York Academy of Sciences, 1094,* 1–12.

Segal, J. (1988). Teachers have enormous power in affecting a child's self-esteem. *Brown University Child Behavior and Development Newsletter, 10,* 1–3.

Seligman, M. E. P. (1990). *Learned optimism: How to change your mind and your life.* New York: Pocket Books.

Seligman, M. E. P. (1995). *The optimistic child.* Boston: Houghton Mifflin.

Shure, M. B. (1996). *Raising a thinking child.* New York: Pocket Books.

Shure, M. B., & Aberson, B. (2013). Enhancing the process of resilience through effective thinking. In S. Goldstein & R. Brooks (Eds.), *Handbook of resilience in children* (2nd ed., pp. 481–503). New York: Springer.

Skinner, E., Pitzer, J., & Steele, J. (2013). Coping as part of motivational resilience in school: A multi-dimensional measure of families, allocations and profiles of academic coping. *Educational and Psychological Measurement, 73,* 803–835.

Taylor, Z. E., & Conger, R. D. (2014). Risk and resilience processes in single mother families: An interactionist perspective. In Z. Sloboda & H. Petras (Eds.), *Defining prevention science* (pp. 195–217). New York: Springer.

Weiner, B. (1974). *Achievement motivation and attribution theory.* Morristown, NJ: General Learning Press.

Werner, E. E. (1993). Risk, resilience, and recovery: Perspectives from the Kauai Longitudinal Study. *Development and Psychopathology, 5,* 503–515.

Werner, E. E., & Smith, R. (2001). *Journeys from childhood to midlife: Risk, resilience, and recovery.* Ithaca, NY: Cornell University Press.

Wright, M. O., Masten, A. S., & Narayan, A. J. (2013). Resilience processes in development: Four waves of research on positive adaptation in the context of adversity. In S. Goldstein & R. Brooks (Eds.), *Handbook of resilience in children* (2nd ed., pp. 15–37). New York: Springer.

Wyman, P. A., Cowen, E. L., Work, W. C., Hoyt-Meyers, L. A., Magnus, K. B., & Fagan, D. B. (1999). Caregiving and developmental factors differentiating young at-risk urban children showing resilient versus stress-affected outcomes: A replication and extension. *Child Development, 709,* 645–659.

Chapter 2

Resilience-Enhancing Factors in Play Therapy

JOHN W. SEYMOUR

In Chapter 1, Brooks and Goldstein have summarized the ways in which resilience research has informed psychotherapy research and practice. The relationship between resilience research and psychotherapy research is both multilayered and interactional. Early resilience research began with descriptive studies identifying the different facets of resilience; subsequent research in this field has evolved into studies on dynamics and processes (Rutter, 1993, 1999, 2007; Wright & Masten, 2006). Psychotherapy research began with descriptions of specific therapeutic models and has shifted in recent years to focus more on the underlying mechanisms shared by all of these models (Prochaska & Norcross, 2010; Saltzman & Norcross, 1990). Masten (2001) has pointed out the strong relationship that resilience research and psychotherapy research share with other areas of child mental health studies, including research in attachment, authoritative parenting, intelligence, self-regulation, self-efficacy, pleasure in mastery, intrinsic motivation, and positive psychology.

Two broad mechanisms affecting resilience are potentially present in the life of every child: risk factors that tend to decrease the development of resilience, and protective factors that tend to enhance its development. Accordingly, the two broad principles of risk reduction and protective enhancement inform the therapeutic processes used by psychotherapists working with children and their families. The questions a child therapist might usefully ask are thus not "How do I do a resilience model?", "How do I incorporate a resilience model with my model?", or even "What products or play materials do I need to buy to do resilience techniques?" The best question for the child therapist is this: "How can the resilience research on these risk and protective factors help me in the process of assessing and treating children and their families?"

Studies in play and play therapy have been greatly enhanced over the past 20 years by interpersonal neurobiology research, which has not only expanded our understanding of interactional mechanisms of child development (Siegel, 2010, 2012), but reinforced the role of natural play as the medium for promoting healthy human development (Brown, 2009; Russ, 2004; Sutton-Smith, 2008). Internal human development is mirrored in the interactions of children through their experiences and relationships, which are commonly mediated through natural play.

In play therapy, the play becomes transformative in providing a child with a new perspective on the self and the environment. Physical activity, personal expression, interpersonal relating, and meaning making with symbols and metaphors in play are all naturally present to some degree in a child's interactive repertoire. Based on these expanded understandings of natural play and child development, the most useful question for today's child therapist is not "Should I include play in my therapy?" or "Should I do play therapy?" It is this: "Since children will bring a rich resource of potential coping skills with them to every session, will I have the awareness, personal availability, and skills to use these natural coping skills effectively to do my best therapeutic work?" Resilience research provides a valuable therapeutic lens through which we can better understand psychotherapy with children, while play therapy is a distinctly well-suited therapeutic method to enhance resilience in children.

RESILIENCE RESEARCH AS A THERAPEUTIC LENS

Early research on resilience was primarily exploratory, describing and cataloging the individual qualities of children who were able to withstand almost any life challenge (Wright & Masten, 2006). This initial understanding of resilience as an internal mechanism rather than an interactional mechanism fueled an unfortunate myth of a near-superhuman "resilient child" able to overcome almost any obstacle. Resilience understood primarily as an internal mechanism can contribute to a naive approach to strength-based approaches, which can seem disrespectful of children's pain and can place undue responsibility on children who seem to be lacking in resilience. Children, with their dependence on their caregivers, sensitivity to others' moods, and magical thinking, can easily feel shamed and blamed with a careless application of a "You can do it!" approach. Crenshaw (2006, 2008) has made a strong case for applying strength-based approaches in ways that do not deny, minimize, or trivialize children's suffering.

Subsequent research on resilience identified it as not so much an individual trait as an interactional process (Rutter, 1987, 1993, 1999, 2007). Resilience as a set of interactional mechanisms (Rutter, 1999; Siegel, 2012) combines a child's individual qualities with an understanding of how these qualities are enhanced or diminished within the social context of family, other support systems, and culture (Benzies & Mychasiuk, 2009; Buckley, Thorngren, & Kleist, 1997; Johnson, 1995; Masten, 2001; Masten & Coatsworth, 1998; Ollendick & Russ, 1999; Rutter, 1999; Wright & Masten, 2006). This interactional approach has been an important factor in applying resilience research to clinical practice (Brooks, 2010; Walsh, 2002, 2003). Through an extensive review of existing resilience studies, Rutter (1999) identified eight resilience mechanisms at work within two broad resilience processes: those reducing risk factors for a child and family, and those increasing the protective factors. Outside the therapy room, the view of resilience as a set of interactive processes has guided public policy and informed community services in promoting optimal child development. Inside the therapy room, it can be equally helpful in guiding the entire therapeutic process. These resilience mechanisms illuminate the dynamics of the child's relationships within the family, as well as the therapeutic relationship. The mechanisms provide specific guidance in assessing the needs and strengths of a child and family, to inform the selection of interventions for both (Goldstein & Brooks, 2006; Seymour, 2010, 2014; Seymour & Erdman, 1996).

PLAY AND THE THERAPEUTIC POWERS OF PLAY

In the Western tradition of psychotherapy, emerging theories and approaches with adults were adapted to address the mental health needs of children. Sigmund Freud saw play as a child's form of free association, providing a look into the inner workings of the child's mind (D'Angelo & Koocher, 2011; Ellenberger, 1981). Anna Freud (1936/1966) and Melanie Klein (1932) each wrote of the important role of play in their psychoanalytic approaches with children. Play was seen as a developmentally appropriate way of interacting with children; it was viewed as providing a natural avenue for establishing the therapeutic relationship, communicating, and problem solving (Donaldson, 1996; O'Connor, 2000). Play was understood not as a separate modality from analysis, but as a seamless part of the therapy process (Winnicott, 1971).

Play includes a certain randomness and uncertainty, allowing opportunities for reinforcing successful ways of relating and problem solving, as well as for expanding a child's personal repertoire of coping skills. Play is a precursor to humans' ability to parent empathically, foster friendships, relate intimately in partnerships, and pursue adult occupations with zest (Slade & Wolf, 1994). Eberle (2014) has put it this way: "Play is an ancient, voluntary, 'emergent' process driven by pleasure that yet strengthens our muscles, instructs our social skills, tempers and deepens our positive emotions, and enables a state of balance that leaves us poised to play some more" (p. 231).

Russ (2004) has identified four broad functions of play that the play therapist enhances in sessions: providing a means of expression for the child; communication and relationship building; insight and working through; and practicing new forms of expression, relating, and problem solving. Studies of play in mammals have demonstrated the importance of play in managing anxiety and developing problem solving related to threats (Siviy, 2010). Sutton-Smith (1997, 2008) has pointed out that humans, as well as certain other mammals, utilize play for the intrinsic value of joy, further contributing to resilience and well-being. In play therapy, the play becomes transformative in providing a new perspective on the self and/or the environment, which is at the heart of resilience as a therapeutic power of play.

RESILIENCE AS A THERAPEUTIC POWER OF PLAY

In the last 20 years, resilience research has informed the practice of play therapy (May, 2006; Seymour, 2010), family play therapy (Seymour & Erdman, 1996), group play therapy (Alvord & Grados, 2005; Alvord, Zucker, & Grados, 2011; Chessor, 2008; Watson, Rich, Sanchez, O'Brien, & Alvord, 2014), and group preventive play (Pedro-Carroll & Jones, 2005). Kazdin (2009), in a review of research on therapeutic processes in child therapy, has pointed out that although there is a wealth of research literature on child psychotherapies, our empirical understanding of processes and outcomes is still limited. He has suggested that the focus needs to be not so much on the choice of model or technique as on the mechanisms of therapeutic change. In play therapy, Schaefer (1993) originally identified 14 change mechanisms common in all therapy models; he has recently expanded the listing to 20 in a coedited book, *The Therapeutic Powers of Play: 20 Core Agents of Change* (Schaefer & Drewes, 2014). This expanded listing includes four categories of therapeutic powers: facilitating communication, fostering emotional wellness, enhancing social relationships, and increasing personal strength. One of the six powers contributing to the fourth category, increasing personal strength, is a newly identified therapeutic power of play: resilience (Schaefer & Drewes, 2014; Seymour, 2014).

APPLYING RESILIENCE
AS A THERAPEUTIC POWER OF PLAY

Brooks (1994a, 1994b) has called for a strong link between resilience research and clinical practice. Resilience research provides a comprehensive and coordinated approach to working with children and their families facing adversity (Tedeschi & Kilmer, 2005). Resilience research can help a play therapist "identify the child's strengths, family and community resources available, and the processes of joining them in reinforcing the child's immediate ability to cope and longer-term ability to be prepared for the next life challenge" (Seymour, 2010, p. 75). In an extensive review of promising practices in child mental health (Simpson, Jivanjee, Koroloff, Doerfler, & García, 2001), four major qualities of successful child mental health services were identified, and all four play a role in the provision of play therapy: coordinated transdisciplinary treatment, a focus on the child's developmental needs, encouragement of family participation in care, and empowerment of family members through strengths and resilience. Rutter's (1999) eight resilience processes provide play therapists with an outline of how to apply play in a therapeutic relationship to enhance resilience in the clients served.

The practice of play therapy and other child psychotherapies has been gradually shifting away from model-specific treatments to more integrated and prescriptive models (Drewes, 2011a, 2011b; Osofsky, 2004). These models focus more on the qualities that establish and maintain the therapeutic relationship, on multimodal methods of assessing children's needs, and on matching these needs with interventions based on an understanding of the therapeutic mechanisms common to most models of child therapy (Shirk & Russell, 1996). Early efforts to define this model have included prescriptive play therapy (Kaduson, Cangelosi, & Schaefer, 1997; Schaefer, 2011), ecosystemic play therapy (O'Connor, 2000), and structured play therapy (Jones, Casado, & Robinson, 2003). Drewes, Bratton, and Schaefer (2011) provide a recent review of these developments, with examples of current integrative play therapy (IPT) practices. As outlined by Drewes (2011a, 2011b), an IPT model is a strength-based approach to play therapy, in which a therapist begins with a focus on the qualities inherent in play that can enhance the therapeutic relationship, selects play therapy interventions that are evidence-based, matches therapeutic interventions to the clients served, and utilizes the therapeutic mechanisms of play therapy (Stien & Kendall, 2004). As an integrative model, it is open to new research developments to inform the practice, and it maintains nimbleness in delivery of care that can be very responsive to changing directions of the child and family (Gil, 2010). The choice of interventions is based on the immediate needs of the child and the child's support system, rather than the outline of a particular theory's model. It allows the therapist to choose between more and less directed approaches, to better match the ebb and flow of the child's ability to sustain the intense feelings and demands of the therapeutic work (Gil, 2006, 2010; Shelby, 2010; Shelby & Felix, 2005). In IPT, the child therapist can implement therapeutic interventions that involve all four of the broad functions of natural play identified by Russ (2004) and mentioned earlier: providing a means of expression for the child; communication and relationship building; insight and working through; and practicing new forms of expression, relating, and problem solving. Rutter's (1999) eight therapeutic mechanisms have recently been updated and applied to play therapy (Seymour, 2014) to describe how resilience acts as a therapeutic power of play:

1. Reducing anxiety and increasing problem solving.
2. Reducing self-blaming.
3. Reducing blaming by others.
4. Reducing isolation and enhancing attachment.
5. Increasing self-esteem and self-efficacy.
6. Increasing creative play to foster creative problem solving.
7. Enhancing nurturing relationships beyond the playroom.
8. Learning to make meaning of life's experiences.

Each of these resilience mechanisms is now explained and illustrated within an IPT model.

Reducing Anxiety and Increasing Problem Solving

Risk factors often have a cascading effect (Rutter, 1999). For instance, children who have experienced intimate-partner violence between their parents may also begin experiencing more worries and losing sleep;

exhibiting more preoccupied behaviors and focusing less on studies; experiencing changes in school and peer relationships; and reducing participation in meaningful activities that enhance their self-efficacy (such as participating in a team sport, sharing a hobby with a family member, or developing a musical talent). The children's personal safety may be at greater risk; mealtimes may be missed; and medical or dental care may be neglected or deferred. Over time, these risk factors take a significant toll. In play therapy, such children exhibit play themes of constant threats from all sides and dilemmas of limited resources and impossible odds. Parent interviews are dominated by an overwhelming list of overlapping emotional, relational, legal, financial, and spiritual stressors.

Play therapy gives these children the opportunity not only to express the anxiety and other feelings resulting from this cascade of effects, but at some point to begin problem solving to reduce some of the risk, identify possible resources, or make some sense of what is happening. The work may be done entirely metaphorically, through play materials, expressive art materials, or a sand tray. Over time, the therapist high-lights themes of solutions or support, fostering a child's own abilities to self-regulate. Any number of play therapy approaches can be used for encouraging nurturing themes for soothing, such as developmen-tally based attachment approaches (Brody, 1997; Jernberg & Booth, 1999; Munns, 2009), expressive and reflective approaches (Crenshaw, 2006, 2010; Green, 2014; Green & Drewes, 2013), or approaches that promote active play for discharging the feelings through appropriate physical means (Jernberg & Booth, 1999; Munns, 2009). Cognitive-behavioral play therapy approaches can also be used, to provide more structure to the process and to make the implicit personal learning more explicit (Drewes, 2006, 2009).

Parents of such children are also experiencing their own cascading risk effects, which may compromise their ability to be helpful to their children or themselves. Parents will need assistance in addressing their own responses to these risk effects, either through referral to another mental health provider or through play therapy approaches that involve the active participation of the parents; such approaches include Thera-play (Jernberg & Booth, 1999; Munns, 2009), family play therapy (Gil, 1994; Schaefer & Carey, 1994; Seymour & Erdman, 1996), and fil-ial therapy (VanFleet, 1994). Therapists should be aware that children, parents, or both may initially experience the referral for counseling and the initiation of the therapeutic relationship more as a new risk than as a benefit. Care should be taken to establish a welcoming and safe environment in the session for all attending. Successful establishment of the therapeutic relationship can then become the first disruption in the cascade of risk and create the foundation of a trusting environment for therapeutic work.

When the cascade of risk extends beyond a child's family and into the community, the therapist will need to attend to continuity of care with other providers serving the child and family (Seymour, 2010). Sometimes the long list of collateral contacts (physician, teacher, school counselor, county social worker, child protective services worker, etc.) becomes daunting for the therapist, but conscientious attention to coordinating care among all parties can have a significant impact on reducing the cascade of risk. Consistently coordinated care contributes to a sense of safety and direction in the therapeutic work for all involved; it extends the influence of the therapeutic alliance well beyond the walls of the therapy room.

Reducing Self-Blaming

Along with reducing risk factors, play therapy can be effective in helping children reduce the self-blaming that often goes along with complex and persistent problems. Clients vary in their baseline sensitivity to environmental risk, and recent research in interpersonal neurobiology has shown that ongoing stress reduces a person's ability to cope with that stress (Barfield, Dobson, Gaskill, & Perry, 2012; Perry, 2006; Perry & Hanbrick, 2008). Children, with their cognitive styles of magical thinking and overestimation of their abilities to modify stress, can develop what O'Connor (2000) has described as a significant distortion of views of causality, leading to a great deal of self-blame.

Children in play therapy may demonstrate play themes of self-blaming or an exaggerated sense of self-responsibility and obligation. If seen in session with siblings, they may play out a caregiving role in the interview process or in play. They may be particularly interested in the well-being of the adults in the room, including the therapist. These are children who have often been labeled as "caregivers" or "parentified children" (Seymour, 2010). Being caregivers, some of these children may not readily respond to nurturing invitations from the therapist; they may even try the role of cotherapist if other family members are present. On the other hand, some of these children may eagerly engage in play and readily accept nurturing invitations, relieved to be able to take a break from their responsible roles.

With such a variety of possible presentations, the play therapist will need to show flexibility in the level of directiveness (Shelby, 2010; Shelby & Felix, 2005) to match the needs of a particular child.

Cognitive-behavioral play therapy strategies can be utilized to address misperceptions of self more directly or to help a child learn desensitization techniques (Drewes, 2009; Knell, 1993, 1994, 1997, 2011).

Reducing Blaming by Others

A child's self-blame is often interpersonally reinforced through blame by others, and sometimes these others have their own exaggerated sense of what a child can or should be responsible for at any given age (Rutter, 1999). Along with the examples of self-blame mentioned above, a child in play may be self-critical or self-deprecating in session. Both in family interviews and in observed play, the therapist may become aware of family patterns of scapegoating particular children. Gil (1994) has described how anxiety can become cyclical between parent and child, with each triggering the other's anxiety, leading to more anxiety-provoking behaviors. This anxiety cycle can amplify a pattern of anger and blame between the child and the parent or other family members.

A therapist using a collaborative, nonjudgmental, strength-based approach to initial interviews can begin the process of disrupting these unfortunate patterns of blame. Parent education on typical child and family development, along with judicious use of reframing problem-focused descriptions to solution-focused descriptions of family life, can help the child and parent begin developing more realistic expectations of their own and others' behaviors.

Parents may benefit from involvement in their own counseling, in family education programs, or in a family-based play therapy approach. In addition, children's self-criticism may be socially reinforced by extended family, teachers, and peers; such children may problem-solve and rehearse through play ways of being more assertive in addressing criticism from these others. Parents may benefit from consultation with the therapist to develop ways of intervening with extended family or others who may contribute to a critical view of their children (Seymour, 2010; Seymour & Erdman, 1996).

Reducing Isolation and Enhancing Attachment

The spiraling processes of increasing risk, self-blame, and blame by others can cause a ripple effect damaging to the child's relationships to caregivers, ranging from temporary disruptions in these relationships to persistent patterns reinforcing already difficult attachment. As the therapeutic relationship is initiated, children will begin to give clues to possible attachment injuries through their interactions with the therapist (and with other family members if these are present). In play therapy, children may present at either end of the engagement continuum—with some being very difficult to engage, and others being engaging to the point of being smothering or controlling to the therapist or others in the room. As sessions begin, some children may socially withdraw and lack any response to the play materials in the room. Others may be hyperactive, impulsive, and even frantic in their use of play materials. The therapist will once again need to be prepared to show a high degree of flexibility to respond successfully to whatever attachment pattern a child presents. Kottman (2011) has described how play therapy rooms, depending on the therapist's preferred model and a child's needs, may range from a "minimalist" approach (a playroom including only basic materials) to a "maximalist" approach (a very well-stocked playroom). Some children may respond best to a well-stocked playroom giving them a lot of diverse opportunities to engage, while others may respond best to a play setting that is less stimulating and more specific to their needs and developmental level, such as in ecosystemic play therapy (O'Connor, 2000).

Crenshaw (2006) has described two levels of engaging children in play therapy, depending on a child's receptiveness and relational abilities: a "coping track" focused on basic supportive care, and an "invitational track" focused on more painful or traumatic work. Many children will spend most of their time in play therapy in the coping track, which will support their strengths and encourage the development of prosocial skills and problem-solving abilities to shore up their adaptive defenses. Children overwhelmed by their experiences will often have an exaggerated fight–flight–freeze response, leading to a reduction in their ability to consider alternative views, take positive actions, or rally personal strengths (Fredrickson, 2001, 2004; Fredrickson & Losada, 2005). In therapeutic play, resilience is built through giving such children opportunities to self-regulate through natural play processes, which will enable them to able connect more effectively with their support systems and develop new strategies for coping.

As with the previous resilience processes, parent–child interventions aimed at calming parents to enable them to connect with and calm their children can be very effective. These include the strategies used in Theraplay with families (Munns, 2000, 2009), family play therapy (Gil, 1994), filial therapy (VanFleet, 1994), and child–parent relationship therapy (Landreth & Bratton, 2006a, 2006b). Likewise, strategies for reducing self-blame enhance not only the earlier-mentioned resilience processes, but this fourth one as well. Coordination of care is yet another resource for reducing isolation, as children and their family members become better acquainted and better connected with helpful resources within their extended families, schools, and communities. Reducing self-blame and reducing the reinforcement of self-blame throughout a child's ecosystem helps to restore and enhance supportive relationships.

Increasing Self-Esteem and Self-Efficacy

Rutter (1999) identified how the negative chain reactions of risk factors can be addressed through positive chain reactions of enhancing protective factors, such as children's sense of self-esteem and self-efficacy. Any early signs of success in addressing life's challenges, whether within or outside therapy sessions, can become building blocks of change. These initial positive experiences bring a feeling of comfort and enjoyment (and, with play, even fun and joy) that becomes self-reinforcing, as these children begin to develop a sense of accomplishment that will prepare them for the next challenge. In session, these children will exhibit varying levels of confidence in exploring the room, trying the play materials, and interacting with the therapist. A child may let the therapist know directly, "I don't do anything good," and leave most leadership of play engagement to the therapist. Beyond the session room, this child may have a very spotty record of involvement in school or leisure enrichment activities.

Brooks (2010) has described how important it is to help children and their families identify "islands of competence" for the children. What are their special interests, talents, and skills that can be encouraged? Highlighting these potential islands of competence in the evaluation and therapeutic process can provide children and family members with places to begin building success. This often begins in the intake process, as a therapist keeps a strong emphasis on a child's strengths. As the therapeutic relationship develops, the child's play in session will begin to suggest particular talents and interests, whether obvious or latent. A child who comes into a session dressed in full athletic uniform or carrying a tuba to play a scale for the therapist obviously suggests some possible islands of competence for development. A child's best courses in school, favorite reading materials, or family interests can also be suggestive. In quieter ways, the therapist will also be able to see signs of a child's particular abilities in displays of curiosity, shows of keen interest in a particular topic, higher-quality interactions with parents and siblings, and the types of play and play materials that are used in sessions.

Increasing Creative Play to Foster Creative Problem Solving

Once children and their families begin to experience some success in the first five resilience processes, the next challenge is supporting them in sustaining these changes and beginning to take the lessons of the sessions into everyday life (Rutter, 1999). Over time, the play therapist will begin to notice a progression in play themes—from earlier themes of repetitive threats and helplessness, to early signs of resourcefulness, hope, and self-agency. Play therapy sessions over time will reflect the ebb and flow of events in a child's life, and the progress and setbacks of the child and family members. Even setbacks can be reframed as opportunities and turning points to help lend a fresh perspective and new energy to the therapeutic process (Seymour & Erdman, 1996; Walsh, 2002, 2003). Themes of play will often shift from a focus on reflecting the presenting problems to rehearsing possible solutions through personal strengths and support systems. As the therapeutic relationship strengthens, it is able to provide the setting and support for children to express their fear and disappointments, and to formulate new efforts at taking therapeutic successes into their lives.

Enhancing Nurturing Relationships beyond the Playroom

To sustain resilience, children need nurturing relationships not only in the session room and in their immediate families, but in their extended support systems (Rutter, 1999). Webb (2007) has recommended that children and family members be assisted in beginning the process of identifying and trusting the positive resources in their families and social settings. Supportive relationships beyond the therapy sessions help to reinforce and sustain the progress that has begun in these sessions. Play themes in sessions will increasingly include helper figures, solutions, and hope when children are finding nurturing beyond the playroom. Play dialogues are often more spontaneous and less stereotyped, with a greater range of affect. Children will often begin to show more leadership in initiating or guiding play, and may become active recruiters to involve any family members present; they may even suggest that other family members be included in future sessions.

Children and family members may benefit from proactive discussions about making wise and balanced choices of enrichment activities and relationships that will provide opportunity and support in developing the children's self-esteem and self-efficacy. In play, children can practice improved skills in finding and maintaining supportive relationships at home, with extended family members, at school, in the community, and with collaborating mental health care providers. In session, the play themes of success and optimism in facing challenges begin to be more evident. Children and family members come to session with reports of new friends made, old friends back in the picture, and enriching activities that begin to show some distance from the negative chain reactions experienced earlier. Brooks (2010) has emphasized the importance of a "charismatic adult" in sustaining a child's resilience. Children need a few strong nurturing relationships with such adults, who can offer stable support and actively encourage the children in implementing the other resilience processes.

Learning to Make Meaning of Life's Experiences

There is growing evidence that for resilience-based growth to be sustained for children and their families, the cognitive and affective processing of experiences is important for reducing risk factors and strengthening the protective factors of self-esteem/self-efficacy and positive relationships (Rutter, 1999). In the early stages of play therapy, a developing play narrative may be less explicitly articulated than identified by patterns in the play, such as a repeating disaster or repeated appearances of protagonist figures. Over time, these themes become more readily spoken, as children narrate their play through theme music, sound effects, and developing word-based narratives. What was once the reflective feedback of the therapist or the discoveries by the child through play begins to inform a story in words as the child makes meaning of these experiences. Early play themes become the source material for stories and metaphors that become transformational for the child, reinforcing strengths and relationships. Cattanach (2008) describes a number of collaborative storytelling approaches to help a child make meaning. As Freeman, Epston, and Lobovits (1997) have shown, problem-saturated stories of family life become transformed into strength-based stories.

This final resilience mechanism is a metaprocess that incorporates all seven of the other processes into a coherent narrative of self and world. Through the creation of a shared narrative, resilience as a therapeutic power of play moves a child from a very private starting point in facing adversity to a more public transition point into the child's beyond-session life. With reduced risk factors and enhanced protective factors, the child faces the world with greater self-confidence, a broadened repertoire of embodied strengths, and stronger bonds with family members and support systems.

CONCLUDING COMMENTS:
RESILIENCE BEYOND THE PLAY THERAPY ROOM

Play therapy sessions provide a safe and creative place for children and their families to develop and enhance qualities of resilience. Rutter's resilience model can provide a practical framework of guidelines for play therapists to integrate the powers of play into their work with children and their families. The resilience research also points therapists to issues of family, community, and culture that can contribute to developing resilience in children (Buckley et al., 1997; Waller, 2001; Wolin & Wolin, 1992, 1993, 1996). These beyond-session factors suggest that play therapists must expand their understanding of therapeutic processes and their therapeutic role to include a role in working with families, consulting with key members of children's support systems, and advocating regarding social problems that contribute to the societal sources of risk. As Masten (2001) has stated, "If major threats to children are those adversities that undermine basic protective systems for development, it follows that efforts to promote competence and resilience in children at risk should focus on strategies that protect or restore the efficacy of these basic systems" (p. 235).

REFERENCES

Alvord, M. K., & Grados, J. J. (2005). Enhancing resilience in children: A proactive approach. *Psychology: Research and Practice, 36*, 238–245.

Alvord, M. K., Zucker, B., & Grados, J. J. (2011). *Resilience builder program for children and adolescents: Enhancing social competence and self-regulation—A cognitive-behavioral group approach.* Champaign, IL: Research Press.

Barfield, S., Dobson, C., Gaskill, R., & Perry, B. D. (2012). Neurosequential model of therapeutics in a therapeutic preschool: Implications for work with children with complex neuropsychiatric problems. *International Journal of Play Therapy, 21*, 30–44.

Benzies, K., & Mychasiuk, R. (2009). Fostering family resiliency: A review of the key protective factors. *Child and Family Social Work, 14*, 103–114.

Brody, V. (1997). *The dialogue of touch: Developmental play therapy* (rev. ed.). Northvale, NJ: Jason Aronson.

Brooks, R. B. (1994a). Children at risk: Fostering resilience and hope. *American Journal of Orthopsychiatry, 64*, 545–553.

Brooks, R. B. (1994b). Diagnostic issues and therapeutic interventions for children at risk. *American Journal of Orthopsychiatry, 64*, 508–509.

Brooks, R. B. (2010). The power of mind-sets: A personal journey to nurture dignity, hope, and resilience in children. In D. A. Crenshaw (Ed.), *Reverence in healing: Honoring strengths without trivializing suffering* (pp. 19–40). Lanham, MD: Jason Aronson.

Brown, S. (2009). *Play: How it shapes the brain, opens the imagination, and invigorates the soul.* New York: Avery.

Buckley, M. R., Thorngren, J. M., & Kleist, D. M. (1997). Family resiliency: A neglected family construct. *Family Journal: Counseling and Therapy for Couples and Families, 5,* 241–246.

Cattanach, A. (2008). *Narrative approaches in play with children.* London: Jessica Kingsley.

Chessor, D. (2008). Developing student wellbeing and resilience using a group process. *Educational and Child Psychology, 25,* 82–90.

Crenshaw, D. A. (2006). *Evocative strategies in child and adolescent psychotherapy.* Lanham, MD: Jason Aronson.

Crenshaw, D. A. (Ed.). (2008). *Child and adolescent psychotherapy: Wounded spirits and healing paths.* Lanham, MD: Jason Aronson.

Crenshaw, D. A. (Ed.). (2010). *Reverence in healing: Honoring strengths without trivializing suffering.* Lanham, MD: Jason Aronson.

D'Angelo, E. J., & Koocher, G. P. (2011). Psychotherapy patients: Children. In J. C. Norcross, G. R. VandenBos, & D. K. Freedheim (Eds.), *History of psychotherapy: Continuity and change* (2nd ed., pp. 430–448). Washington, DC: American Psychological Association.

Donaldson, G. (1996). Between practice and theory: Melanie Klein, Anna Freud, and the development of child analysis. *Journal of the History of the Behavioral Sciences, 32,* 160–176.

Drewes, A. A. (2006). Play-based interventions. *Journal of Early Childhood and Infant Psychology, 2,* 139–156.

Drewes, A. A. (2009). *Blending play therapy with cognitive behavioral therapy: Evidence-based and other effective treatments and techniques.* Hoboken, NJ: Wiley.

Drewes, A. A. (2011a). Integrating play therapy theories into practice. In A. A. Drewes, S. C. Bratton, & C. E. Schaefer (Eds.), *Integrative play therapy* (pp. 21–35). Hoboken, NJ: Wiley.

Drewes, A. A. (2011b). Integrative play therapy. In C. E. Schaefer (Ed.), *Foundations of play therapy* (2nd ed., pp. 349–364). Hoboken, NJ: Wiley.

Drewes, A. A., Bratton, S. C., & Schaefer, C. E. (Eds.). (2011). *Integrative play therapy.* Hoboken, NJ: Wiley.

Eberle, S. G. (2014). The elements of play: Toward a philosophy and a definition of play. *American Journal of Play, 6,* 214–233.

Ellenberger, H. F. (1981). *The discovery of the unconscious: The history and evolution of dynamic psychiatry.* New York: Basic Books.

Fredrickson, B. L. (2001). The role of positive emotions in positive psychology: The broaden-and-build theory of positive emotions. *American Psychologist, 56,* 218–226.

Fredrickson, B. L. (2004). The broaden-and-build theory of positive emotions. *Philosophical Transactions of the Royal Society of London: Series B. Biological Sciences, 359,* 1367–1377.

Fredrickson, B. L., & Losada, M. F. (2005). Positive affect and the complex dynamics of human flourishing. *American Psychologist, 60,* 678–686.

Freeman, J., Epston, D., & Lobovits, D. (1997). *Playful approaches to serious problems: Narrative therapy with children and their families.* New York: Norton.

Freud, A. (1966). *The ego and the mechanisms of defense* (rev. ed.). New York: International Universities Press. (Original work published 1936)

Gil, E. (1994). *Play in family therapy.* New York: Guilford Press.

Gil, E. (2006). *Helping abused and traumatized children: Integrating directive and nondirective approaches.* New York: Guilford Press.

Gil, E. (Ed.). (2010). *Working with children to heal interpersonal trauma: The power of play.* New York: Guilford Press.

Goldstein, S., & Brooks, R. B. (Eds.). (2006). *Handbook of resilience in children.* New York: Springer.

Green, E. J. (2014). *The handbook of Jungian play therapy with children and adolescents.* Baltimore: Johns Hopkins University Press.

Green, E. J., & Drewes, A. (Eds.). (2013). *Integrating expressive arts and play therapy with children: A guidebook for clinicians and educators.* Hoboken, NJ: Wiley.

Jernberg, A., & Booth, P. (1999). *Theraplay* (2nd ed.). San Francisco: Jossey-Bass.

Johnson, A. C. (1995). Resiliency mechanisms in culturally diverse families. *Family Journal: Counseling and Therapy for Couples and Families, 3,* 316–324.

Jones, K. D., Casado, M., & Robinson, E. H. (2003). Structured play therapy: A model for choosing topics and activities. *International Journal of Play Therapy, 12,* 31–47.

Kaduson, H. G., Cangelosi, D., & Schaefer, C. E. (Eds.). (1997). *The playing cure: Individualized play therapy for specific childhood problems.* Northvale, NJ: Jason Aronson.

Kazdin, A. E. (2009). Understanding how and why psychotherapy leads to change. *Psychotherapy Research, 19,* 418–428.

Kottman, T. (2011). *Play therapy: Basics and beyond* (2nd ed.). Alexandria, VA: American Counseling Association.

Klein, M. (1932). *The psycho-analysis of children.* London: Hogarth Press.

Knell, S. (1993). *Cognitive-behavioral play therapy.* Northvale, NJ: Jason Aronson.

Knell, S. (1994). Cognitive-behavioral play therapy. In K. J. O'Connor & C. E. Schaefer (Eds.), *Handbook of play therapy* (Vol. 2, pp. 111–142). New York: Wiley.

Knell, S. (1997). Cognitive-behavioral play therapy. In K. J. O'Connor & L. M. Braverman (Eds.), *Play therapy theory and practice: A comparative presentation* (pp. 79–99). New York: Wiley.

Knell, S. M. (2011). Cognitive-behavioral play therapy. In C. E. Schaefer (Ed.), *Foundations of play therapy* (2nd ed., pp. 313–328). Hoboken, NJ: Wiley.

Landreth, G. L., & Bratton, S. C. (2006a). *Child parent relationship therapy (CPRT): A 10-session filial therapy model.* New York: Routledge.

Landreth, G. L., & Bratton, S. C. (2006b). *Child parent relationship therapy (CPRT): Treatment manual.* New York: Routledge.

Masten, A. S. (2001). Ordinary magic: Resilience processes in development. *American Psychologist, 56,* 227–238.

Masten, A. S., & Coatsworth, J. D. (1998). The development of competence in favorable and unfavorable environments: Lessons from research on successful children. *American Psychologist, 53,* 205–220.

May, D. (2006). Time-limited play therapy to enhance resiliency in children. In C.

E. Schaefer & H. G. Kaduson (Eds.), *Contemporary play therapy: Theory, research, and practice* (pp. 293–306). New York: Guilford Press.

Munns, E. (2000). *Theraplay: Innovations in attachment-enhancing play therapy.* Northvale, NJ: Jason Aronson.

Munns, E. (Ed.). (2009). *Applications of family and group Theraplay.* Lanham, MD: Jason Aronson.

O'Connor, K. J. (2000). *Play therapy primer* (2nd ed.). New York: Wiley.

Ollendick, T., & Russ, S. (1999). Psychotherapy with children and families: Historical Traditions and current trends. In S. Russ & T. Ollendick (Eds.), *Handbook of psychotherapy with children and families* (pp. 3–13). New York: Kluwer Academic Press/Plenum Press.

Osofsky, J. D. (Ed.). (2004). *Young children and trauma: Intervention and treatment.* New York: Guilford Press.

Pedro-Carroll, J., & Jones, S. H. (2005). A preventive play intervention to foster children's resilience in the aftermath of divorce. In L. A. Reddy, T. M. Files-Hall, & C. E. Schaefer (Eds.), *Empirically based play interventions for children* (pp. 51–75). Washington, DC: American Psychological Association.

Perry, B. D. (2006). The neurosequential model of therapeutics: Applying principles of neuroscience to clinical work with traumatized and maltreated children. In N. B. Webb (Ed.), *Working with traumatized youth in child welfare* (pp. 27–52). New York: Guilford Press.

Perry, B. D., & Hanbrick, E. P. (2008). The neurosequential model of therapeutics. *Reclaiming Children and Youth, 17,* 38–43.

Prochaska, J. O., & Norcross, J. C. (2010). *Systems of psychotherapy: A transtheoretical analysis* (7th ed.). Belmont, CA: Brooks/Cole.

Russ, S. W. (2004). *Play in child development and psychotherapy: Toward empirically supported practice.* Mahwah, NJ: Erlbaum.

Rutter, M. E. (1987). Psychosocial resilience and protective mechanisms. *American Journal of Orthopsychiatry, 57,* 316–331.

Rutter, M. E. (1993). Resilience: Some conceptual considerations. *Journal of Adolescent Health, 14,* 626–631.

Rutter, M. E. (1999). Resilience concepts and findings: Implications for family therapy. *Journal of Family Therapy, 21,* 119–144.

Rutter, M. E. (2007). Resilience, competence, and coping. *Child Abuse and Neglect, 31,* 205–209.

Saltzman, N., & Norcross, J. C. (1990). *Therapy wars: Contention and convergence in differing clinical approaches.* San Francisco: Jossey-Bass.

Schaefer, C. E. (Ed.). (1993). *The therapeutic powers of play.* Northvale, NJ: Jason Aronson.

Schaefer, C. E. (2011). Prescriptive play therapy. In C. E. Schaefer (Ed.), *Foundations of play therapy* (2nd ed., pp. 365–378). Hoboken, NJ: Wiley.

Schaefer, C. E., & Carey, L. J. (Eds.). (1994). *Family play therapy.* Northvale, NJ: Jason Aronson.

Schaefer, C. E., & Drewes, A. A. (Eds.). (2014). *The therapeutic powers of play: 20 core agents of change* (2nd ed.). Hoboken, NJ: Wiley.

Seymour, J. W. (2010). Resiliency-based approaches and the healing process in play therapy. In D. A. Crenshaw (Ed.), *Reverence in healing: Honoring strengths without trivializing suffering* (pp. 71–84). Lanham, MD: Jason Aronson.

Seymour, J. W. (2014). Resiliency as a therapeutic power of play. In C. E. Schaefer & A. A. Drewes (Eds.), *The therapeutic powers of play: 20 core agents of change* (2nd ed., pp. 241–263). Hoboken, NJ: Wiley.

Seymour, J. W., & Erdman, P. E. (1996). Family play therapy using a resiliency model. *International Journal of Play Therapy, 5*, 19–30.

Shelby, J. S. (2010). Cognitive-behavioral therapy and play therapy for childhood trauma and loss. In N. B. Webb (Ed.), *Helping bereaved children: A handbook for practitioners* (3rd ed., pp. 263–277). New York: Guilford Press.

Shelby, J. S., & Felix, E. D. (2005). Posttraumatic play therapy: The need for an integrated model of directive and nondirective approaches. In L. A. Reddy, T. M. Files-Hall, & C. E. Schaefer (Eds.), *Empirically based play interventions for children* (pp. 79–103). Washington, DC: American Psychological Association.

Shirk, S. R., & Russell, R. L. (1996). *Change processes in child psychotherapy: Revitalizing treatment and research.* New York: Guilford Press.

Siegel, D. J. (2010). *Mindsight: The new science of personal transformation.* New York: Random House.

Siegel, D. J. (2012). *The developing mind: How relationships and the brain interact to shape who we are* (2nd ed.). New York: Guilford Press.

Simpson, J., Jivanjee, P., Koroloff, N., Doerfler, A., & Garcia, M. (2001). *Systems of care: Promising practices in children's mental health: Vol. 3. Promising practices in early childhood mental health.* Washington, DC: Center for Effective Collaboration and Practice, American Institutes for Research.

Siviy, S. M. (2010). Play and adversity: How the playful mammalian brain withstands threats and anxieties. *American Journal of Play, 2*, 297–314.

Slade, A., & Wolf, D. E. (Eds.). (1994). *Children at play: Clinical and developmental approaches to meaning and representation.* New York: Oxford University Press.

Stien, P. T., & Kendall, J. (2004). *Psychological trauma and the developing brain: Neurologically based interventions for troubled children.* New York: Haworth Press.

Sutton-Smith, B. (1997). *The ambiguity of play.* Cambridge, MA: Harvard University Press.

Sutton-Smith, B. (2008). Play theory: A personal journey and new thoughts. *American Journal of Play, 1*, 82–125.

Tedeschi, R. G., & Kilmer, R. P. (2005). Assessing strengths, resilience, and growth to guide clinical interventions. *Professional Psychology: Research and Practice, 36*, 230–237.

VanFleet, R. (1994). *Filial Therapy: Strengthening parent–child relationships through play.* Sarasota, FL: Professional Resource Press.

Waller, M. A. (2001). Resilience in ecosystemic context: Evolution of the concept. *American Journal of Orthopsychiatry, 71*, 290–297.

Walsh, F. (2002). A family resilience framework: Innovative practice application. *Family Relations, 51*, 130–137.

Walsh, F. (2003). Family resilience: Strengths forged through adversity. In F. Walsh (Ed.), *Normal family processes: Growing diversity and complexity* (pp. 399–423). New York: Guilford Press.

Watson, C. C., Rich, B. A., Sanchez, L., O'Brien, K., & Alvord, M. K. (2014). Preliminary study of resilience-based group therapy for improving the functioning of anxious children. *Child and Youth Care Forum, 43*, 269–286.

Webb, N. B. (Ed.). (2007). *Play therapy with children in crisis: A casebook for practitioners* (3rd ed.). New York: Guilford Press.

Winnicott, D. W. (1971). *Playing and reality.* London: Tavistock.

Wolin, S., & Wolin, S. J. (1996). The challenge model: Working with the strengths of children of substance abusing parents. *Child and Adolescent Psychiatric Clinics of North America, 5*(1), 243–256.

Wolin, S. J., & Wolin, S. (1992). The challenge model: How children rise above adversity. *Family Dynamics of Addiction Quarterly, 2*(2), 10–22.

Wolin, S. J., & Wolin, S. (1993). *The resilient self: How survivors of troubled families rise above adversity.* New York: Villard Books.

Wright, M. O., & Masten, A. S. (2006). Resilience processes in development. In S. Goldstein & R. B. Brooks (Eds.), *Handbook of resilience in children* (pp. 17–38). New York: Springer.

Part II

CLINICAL APPLICATIONS

Chapter 3

The Use of Metaphors and Storytelling Techniques to Nurture Resilience in Children

ROBERT BROOKS
SUZANNE BROOKS

The application of storytelling and metaphors, including the use of bibliotherapy, has a rich history within the domain of play therapy with children. Many different therapeutic approaches have included storytelling and metaphors, with each inviting varying degrees of structure and input on the part of the therapist (Berg-Cross & Berg-Cross, 1976; Brooks, 1981, 1985, 1987; Crenshaw, 2006, 2008b, 2010; Drewes, 2014; Frey, 1993; Gardner, 1971, 1972, 1975; Gil, 2014; Goldings, 1974; Malchiodi & Crenshaw, 2014; Mills & Crowley, 1986, 2014; Nickerson, 1975; Robertson & Barford, 1970; Schaefer & Cangelosi, 1993; Schaefer & Drewes, 2014).

In this chapter, we review and offer illustrations of the use of storytelling and metaphors to develop a trusting relationship with and nurture resilience in child patients—a process that begins during the first session. Our view of resilience is guided by the concept of a "resilient mindset" articulated by Brooks and Goldstein (Brooks, 2010; Brooks & Brooks, 2014; Brooks & Goldstein, 2001, 2007, 2011, and Chapter 1, this volume). Others have also developed their therapeutic goals and activities in play therapy within a resilience-based model (Crenshaw,

2008a, 2010; Seymour, 2010, 2014, and Chapter 2, this volume; Seymour & Erdman, 1996).

Before we describe our application of storytelling and metaphors, we very briefly spotlight the two guiding principles involved in a resilience-based approach that have been noted by Brooks and Goldstein in Chapter 1 of this volume. The first pertains to the impact of the relationship that the therapist develops with the patient; the second involves the components of a resilient mindset, which serve as guideposts for our therapeutic journey.

THE CHILD THERAPIST
AS A CHARISMATIC ADULT

In searching for effective techniques to use with children, clinicians must never lose sight of a primary goal: establishing a positive relationship with a child. In the absence of such a relationship, any therapeutic strategies are likely to be compromised and to prove ineffective. As we have often said, "Children don't care what you know until they first know you care." It is our belief that the therapist–child relationship can initially be nurtured via storytelling and metaphors, and that once this relationship is solidified, these same techniques can be employed to continue to help the child confront his/her struggles.

Brooks and Goldstein (2001, 2007, and Chapter 1, this volume) have emphasized the power of the therapeutic relationship. In Chapter 1, they cite the late psychologist Julius Segal's observation of a basic research finding about resilience in children: "One factor turns out to be the presence in their lives of a *charismatic adult*—a person with whom they can identify and from whom they gather strength" (p. 3). We believe that an essential therapeutic goal is for clinicians to strive to assume the role of a charismatic adult for their patients. To adopt this role, therapists must subscribe to the belief that their interventions can assist children to become increasingly hopeful and resilient. Brooks and Goldstein propose two questions in Chapter 1 for therapists to ask themselves: "At the end of each therapy session, is my patient stronger because of things I've said or done or is my patient less strong and hopeful? Has my patient gathered strength from me?"

Therapists, in explaining the notion of charismatic adult to the child's parents and/or teachers, should prompt these caregivers to consider similar questions: "When I put my children to bed at night, do I ask, 'Are my son and daughter stronger because of things I've said or done today or are they less strong? Have they gathered strength from me?'"

"At the end of the school day, do I as a teacher ask, 'Are all of the students in my classroom stronger because of things I've said or done today or are they less strong? Have they gathered strength from me?' "

In our experience, the image of a charismatic adult is quickly adopted by concerned adults—as was illustrated when one set of parents said, "We really want our child to see us as charismatic adults," and when a principal of a middle school asserted, "All staff and faculty in this school aim to be charismatic adults. We constantly refer to this image at our staff meetings." Again, child therapists should always strive to serve in that role in the lives of their patients.

THE CHARACTERISTICS
OF A RESILIENT MINDSET

It can be a challenge for us as child therapists to answer the questions about whether children have gathered strength from us, especially since the concept of "strength" and its measurement are far from precise. The concept of a resilient mindset proposed by Brooks and Goldstein (2001 and Chapter 1, this volume) offers a framework for examining the outlook and skills associated with strength and resilience. Chapter 1 lists the characteristics of a resilient mindset. Resilient children:

- Feel loved and accepted.
- Have learned to set realistic goals and expectations and goals for themselves.
- Are able to define the aspects of their lives over which they have control and to focus their energy and attention on those, rather than on factors over which they have little, if any, influence.
- Believe that they have the ability to solve problems and make informed decisions.
- Take realistic credit for their successes and achievements but acknowledge the input and support of adults for these successes.
- View mistakes, setbacks, and obstacles as challenges to confront and master rather than as stressors to avoid.
- Recognize and accept their vulnerabilities and weaknesses, seeing these as areas for improvement, rather than as unchangeable flaws.
- Recognize, enjoy, and use their strengths, or what we call their "islands of competence."
- Feel comfortable with and relate well to both peers and adults.
- Believe that they make a positive difference in the lives of others.

We now turn to the ways in which storytelling and metaphors can facilitate the therapeutic goal of nurturing the components of this mindset in our patients.

THE THERAPEUTIC IMPACT
OF STORYTELLING AND METAPHORS

While this chapter pertains to therapy with children, the use of storytelling and metaphors also holds a prominent position in therapy with adults (Barker, 1985; Gordon, 1978; Kopp, 1995; Lankton & Lankton, 1989; White & Epston, 1990). The brilliance of psychiatrist Milton Erickson was often captured by the ways in which he communicated therapeutic messages via stories and metaphors (Dolan, 1985; Mills & Crowley, 2014; Zeig, 1980).

One might question why storytelling and metaphors have found such a welcoming place in the world of therapy with both children and adults. I (Robert Brooks) was once asked at a child therapy workshop I was conducting, "Why can't we just communicate directly with our child patients? Why do we have to disguise the message through stories and metaphors? Why not use real-life, direct messages?" I responded:

> "We should always be searching for the most effective ways of communicating with our patients so that they can benefit from our interventions. Sometimes children will be more willing to listen to our messages if we communicate through stories and metaphors. And it's not unusual for children themselves to introduce stories and metaphors without prompting. I think a key question to ask is, 'How best do I communicate with children in therapy so that I help them to understand their emotions and thoughts and to cope more effectively with the challenges they face?'"

I emphasized that the answer will vary not only from one child to the next, but even from one session to the next for the same child.

Richard Gardner, a renowned psychiatrist who developed the "Mutual Storytelling" technique, wrote numerous therapeutic books for children, and designed several popular therapeutic board games (Gardner, 1971, 1972, 1975), offered the following observation about the power of storytelling in therapy:

> This approach employs one of the most ancient and powerful methods of communication. The fable, the legend, and the myth have proved

universally appealing and potent vehicles for transmitting insights, values, and standards of behavior. The child is spared the anxiety he might experience with more direct attempts to impart or elicit conscious insights. One could say that the interpretations bypass the conscious, appeal to and are received by the unconscious. Direct verbalization, confrontation, and interpretation—so reminiscent of parents and teachers—are avoided. Psychoanalytic interpretations, often too alien for the child's comprehension, need not be employed. (1993, p. 200)

Although we concur with Gardner's viewpoint, we would emphasize that storytelling not only allows children to learn, absorb, and apply insights about their internal and external worlds, but also provides them with a rich means for sharing these worlds with others. In addition, messages conveyed via stories appear to be more easily recalled and utilized by both children and adults, even years after the initial telling of a story. On numerous occasions, I have heard the following kind of message from participants who were attending one of my workshops, "I heard you 10 years ago. Are you going to tell the story of [the person mentions the story]? I found your story very helpful, and it reminded me of different ways of looking at and responding to situations."

Although "metaphors" constitute a separate concept from "storytelling," the two concepts are certainly similar in many respects and are often intertwined. Kopp (1971) defined "metaphor" as "a way of speaking in which one thing is expressed in terms of another, whereby this bringing together throws new light on the character of what is being described" (p. 17). Gordon (1978), referring to therapy with adults—although his remarks are just as relevant to child therapy—wrote, "All therapeutic approaches and systems make explicit and implicit use of metaphors" (p. 8).

Mills and Crowley (1986) eloquently expressed their understanding of metaphors when they observed:

Metaphor is a form of symbolic language that has been used for centuries as a method of teaching in many fields. The parables of the Old and New Testaments, the holy writings of the Kabbalah, the koans of Zen Buddhism, the allegories of literature, the images of poetry, and the fairy tales of storytellers—all make use of metaphor to convey an idea in an indirect yet paradoxically more meaningful way. Recognition of this special power of the metaphor has also been grasped by every parent and grandparent who, observing the forlorn features of the young child, seek to bring consolation and nurturance by relating an experience to which the child can intuitively relate. (p. 7)

Gil (2014) recently wrote that while the concept of metaphor has been defined in different ways, there is a commonality among the definitions: "It is usually considered something that is used to present something else, a symbol" (p. 160). She credits the work of Erickson (see, e.g., Erickson & Rossi, 1979) for calling awareness to the power of metaphor in therapeutic endeavors. Gil has articulated guidelines for the application of metaphors in child therapy, expressing the following viewpoint:

> Whether the metaphors are initiated by clients or their clinicians, they serve as projections or representations of something that cannot always be acknowledged or verbalized. . . . Metaphors also offer opportunities for healing through processing of difficult experiences. . . . An integrative approach allows for processing the metaphors both symbolically and verbally; therapists help children to externalize their thoughts and feelings by staying within their metaphors, rather than drawing too-quick correlations between the metaphor and real life. In fact, if children were feeling able or willing to speak about their distress, they would do so. Instead they seem to find it much easier to "speak" through metaphor. (pp. 175–176)

Ekstein (1970) discussed his work with children with borderline symptoms, especially a technique he labeled "interpretation within the metaphor." He stated:

> If the metaphoric mode chosen by the borderline child is responded to correctly, the danger of possibly arousing the pre-existing paranoid trends is eliminated. In addition, he cannot help but know what the therapist is getting at, and, furthermore, feel safe because he also knows that he is not going to be forced to reveal or deal with anything except that which he himself selects. (p. 162)

The nature of Milton Erickson's clinical interventions, cited by Gil (2014) as a major influence in the area of therapeutic metaphors, was captured by Haley (1973) as follows:

> In the way he listens to and observes a subject, as well as the way he responds, he deals with the multiple metaphoric messages that are constantly communicated between people in their interchange. . . . Although Erickson communicates with patients in metaphor, what clearly distinguishes him from other therapists is his unwillingness to interpret to people what metaphors mean. He does not translate "unconscious" communication into conscious form. Whatever the patient says in metaphoric form Erickson responds [to] in kind. By parables, by interpersonal action, and by directives, he works within

the metaphor to bring about change. He seems to feel that the depth and swiftness of the change can be prevented if the person suffers a translation in the communication. (pp. 27–29)

Ekstein's and Erickson's positions raise an interesting question that has been posed by many clinicians: How aware should a child be made of the parallels between a metaphor or story and what is transpiring in the child's real life? In addressing this issue, Brooks (1985) noted:

> While the question of whether or not the patient is aware of the meaning of metaphors produced in therapy is important, it seems secondary to the challenge for the therapist of selecting those metaphors that will have special meaning for and positive impact on the patient. Preferentially, the metaphors should be those first used by the patient, but a therapist tuned into a patient's inner world can introduce metaphors that will immediately communicate a rich level of understanding. . . . The therapist's use of particular metaphors should not be seen as mutually exclusive from seemingly more direct, less symbolic forms of communication; both forms of communication involve intertwining threads that contribute to the richness of the therapeutic fabric. (p. 765)

ELICITING STORIES AND METAPHORS DURING THE DIAGNOSTIC PHASE

Metaphors and stories are often available during the first meeting with a child. They serve not only as a source of information about the child's inner world and struggles, but as a vehicle through which the therapist can begin to assist the child to engage in the therapeutic process and become more resilient. As one example, clinicians who make use of projective tests such as the Rorschach or thematic cards have a resource through which to actively invite the emergence of metaphors and stories.

Clinical Case Example: The Bat with Holes in It

I (Robert Brooks) have advocated, when indicated, the modification of the standard administration of projective tests in the service of identifying key issues in a child's life that may then be used in therapy (Brooks, 1983). An example of this flexibility in test administration involved a 9-year-old boy whose leg was deformed because of a car accident that occurred when he was a toddler. To the first Rorschach card he saw, he responded, "A bat with holes in it." Given that diagnostic questions about this child related to issues of self-esteem, body image, relationship with peers and adults, and coping style, I posed several questions about this response:

"What is the bat doing?"
"How did the bat get the holes?"
"How did the bat feel about having holes?"
"Do the holes keep the bat from doing certain things?"
"What do other bats feel about this bat?"
"Can anyone help the bat?"
"Can the bat ask anyone for help?"

Answers to these questions provided me with information to initiate a therapeutic story, with the boy's input. The story and metaphors concerned a bat that was helped to face adversity and cope more effectively with his struggles, despite the presence of holes on his body. Given the boy's responses to my questions, it became evident that the bat was a representation of himself.

Some professionals, while not denying that significant information can be garnered by modifying standard administration procedures, have posed another important question: "Would it be more advantageous to administer tests in a standardized way first, and then return to ask particular questions for elaboration?" There is certainly validity to following this approach, but we would argue that sometimes, if a clinician does not ask certain questions immediately following a child's response, the emotions and thoughts surrounding the response are lost and their richness is reduced.

We are not advocating a chaotic approach to diagnostic interviewing and testing, or implying that norms are irrelevant. Rather, as Korchin (1976) has observed,

> The clinician must be sensitive, ingenious, and inventive. It is sometimes necessary to improvise new procedures or alter standard tests even on the spur of the moment. . . . Variation from standard procedure means, of course, that available norms may be inapplicable. However, the gain in personologically useful information can offset the loss of standardization and norms. (p. 210)

Clinical Case Example: The Dying Brain and the Flow of Worried Thoughts

I (Suzanne Brooks) have often found diagnostic testing to be very useful to identify the metaphors of children that represent their emotional strengths and vulnerabilities. For example, Katie, an intellectually precocious 9-year-old girl, was referred to me with extreme anxiety, difficulties producing written work in school, and distractibility. During the first session, Katie offered a very powerful and concerning statement regarding how it felt to experience such anxiety. She said, "Sometimes I felt I wanted to die."

Katie quickly qualified this by saying she did not want to die; rather, she wanted her "brain to die." When I queried further, Katie provided a metaphor that would be used in assisting her to confront her struggles. She explained that her "worried thoughts flowed so fast" that she wasn't able to get them to go away. She then told me she was hopeful that the testing would give her and her parents and teachers ideas to help with her problems.

There were several noteworthy observations from the testing that paralleled Katie's assertion that her "worried thoughts flowed so fast." She became easily stressed, which, not surprisingly, impaired her performance on cognitive, intellectual, and personality tests. Specifically, when Katie was stressed, she rushed through tasks, frequently changed her responses, and had difficulty maintaining focus on relevant information.

I made use of the metaphors of the "brain dying" and "worried thoughts flowing so fast" not only to explain the test results to Katie, but also to convey that these were problems that could be addressed. Using information gathered from intellectual and projective testing, I explained to Katie that her mind not only thought very quickly, but thought about many things at once—a situation that added to her worries. I then reframed Katie's two images by saying that her brain worked very well in many ways, but that kids who work very quickly need to teach their brains to "put on the brakes." This last statement was introduced to convey the belief that there were solutions to Katie's problems—to begin the process of nurturing hope and resilience.

Katie was intrigued by the notion of "putting on the brakes" and asked me how that might be accomplished. I, continuing to reference Katie's metaphors, began a dialogue that was to continue in future sessions. I talked about the tools that can help to slow kids' brains down, such as using graphic organizers, putting worried thoughts in a box and referring to them later, and taking physical breaks when their brains start moving too fast.

I also told Katie that I would share these ideas with her parents and teachers, so they could implement similar strategies at home and school. Katie quickly began referencing "putting on the brakes" and "slowing down my brain"—images that proved extremely useful in all parts of her life. The metaphors served as representations for Katie that she possessed problem-solving skills and could begin to control her worrisome, fast thoughts—two essential features of a resilient mindset.

Obviously, whether or not a clinician uses structured psychological tests or interview questions, the clinician's initial meetings with a child provide fertile ground for identifying the child's "story" and the metaphors that help to symbolize that story. They also provide opportunities to begin to develop an alliance with the child and inform the child about the therapeutic process.

THE INITIAL SESSIONS OF THERAPY: MESSAGES AND METAPHORS

Regardless of their theoretical outlook, most if not all clinicians would include the establishment of a therapeutic alliance as the major goal of the beginning of therapy (Brooks, 1985; Keith, 1968). An alliance, which must be nurtured throughout therapy, involves trust and cooperation between patient and therapist and is rooted in the patient's feeling safe, secure, and free from being judged or criticized. The personal characteristics of therapists, including their warmth, empathy, and caring, are vital and essential ingredients of alliance building. However, we believe that the alliance can be enhanced by the messages that therapists communicate directly or through metaphors and stories to enlighten patients about the treatment process.

There are several key messages a therapist should consider introducing during the first few sessions with a child and reinforcing in subsequent meetings (Brooks, 1985). These messages pertain to the following interrelated goals: (1) to identify and articulate the issues or problems that brought the child to therapy; (2) to develop the image of the therapist as someone who can help ease the problems the child is facing; (3) to advance the notion that problems can be solved in therapy; (4) to highlight the belief that solving problems involves a mutual effort between child and therapist (as well as the involvement of significant others, such as parents and teachers); (5) to emphasize that the child is an active participant in therapy; and (6) to acknowledge that setbacks may occur and that problems may reemerge, but that such setbacks can serve as sources of information for developing new coping strategies for future success.

These messages serve to create the portrait of the therapist as a charismatic adult in the child's life—as a person from whom the child can gather strength. The messages also involve strengthening several vital features of a resilient mindset, including the belief that we all are or can become "the authors of our own lives." An acceptance of this authorship is associated with being proactive rather than reactive, coping effectively with setbacks, and developing a more optimistic outlook (Brooks & Goldstein, 2001, 2004).

To help a child move beyond a feeling of helplessness and avoid assuming a victim's mentality, and to initiate steps to improve the child's life, are significant therapeutic goals. Changing the child's beliefs about and perceptions of both success and failure in his/her life is an important dimension of self-esteem and resilience (Brooks, 1984; Brooks & Goldstein, 2001; Weiner, 1974). We must help child patients recognize that when conditions improve in their lives, they have contributed to this improvement. And when setbacks occur, we must help them learn from these setbacks that they can become effective problem solvers in their future activities (Shure, 1996; Shure & Aberson, 2013).

I (Robert Brooks) recall Steven, a boy I saw in therapy for 2 years. In one of our last sessions, Steven expressed this strength-based outlook. He said that he hoped I would not be offended by what he was about to say. Steven told me that I had been very helpful to him, but without his (Steven's) "hard work and effort, none of the achievements would have been possible." I replied that not only was I not offended by his statement, but, if anything, he had just verbalized what any therapist would wish to hear.

As noted above, it is our experience that children provide therapists with opportunities during the first few sessions to orient them to therapeutic tasks and goals, but that these opportunities are often clothed in metaphors and stories. While each patient's metaphors are uniquely rooted in his or her own histories and may contain various meanings, we recommend that during the initial phase of treatment the therapist use the metaphors that are produced to educate the patient about the therapeutic process, to reinforce the therapeutic alliance, and to begin the process of nurturing a resilient mindset. Such a selective response should not be seen as ignoring other meanings of the metaphors; rather, these other possible meanings should be registered and stored by the therapist to be used, when indicated, in future sessions.

The following two case examples involve children seen by me (Robert Brooks). Both represent the ways in which a child's metaphors were applied in the beginning sessions of therapy. In both instances, the metaphors of the initial sessions provided information that was used in the creation of stories in later sessions. The cases are presented largely in dialogue format, to allow us to share the rationales and goals behind my statements more easily.

Clinical Case Example: Don't Push on a Grasshopper

Meredith, a 6-year-old girl, was referred because of oppositional behavior and temper tantrums. During the first session she informed me that she liked grasshoppers, adding, "You have to treat them nicely and not press on them too hard, or they won't feel like jumping."

As might seem apparent, I interpreted her warning about how to treat grasshoppers as a message about how she expected me to relate to her. She appeared to be expressing that if I attempted to push her too vigorously, she would refuse to cooperate with me. Accordingly, I responded in the following manner:

> DR. BROOKS: Do grasshoppers want to learn to jump? [This was intended to assess her wish to learn and grow.]
>
> MEREDITH: Yes.
>
> DR. BROOKS: Do they need help in learning to jump? [I wanted to assess whether she felt others could be helpful.]
>
> MEREDITH: Yes.
>
> DR. BROOKS: Who can help them?
>
> MEREDITH: The trainer [an apparent therapist figure].
>
> DR. BROOKS: How does the trainer do that?
>
> MEREDITH: He pushes them.
>
> DR. BROOKS: Does he ever push them too hard? [This was based on Meredith's initial comment.]
>
> MEREDITH: Sometimes.
>
> DR. BROOKS: Why? [I was trying to determine whether she experienced the pushing too hard as an intentional and/or angry act.]
>
> MEREDITH: I don't know.
>
> DR. BROOKS: Do you think the trainer wants to push down too hard on the grasshopper?
>
> MEREDITH: Some trainers might. Some trainers are mean. ["Mean" was a word Meredith used to describe her teacher, a woman whom Meredith did not like.]
>
> DR. BROOKS: How come?
>
> MEREDITH: I'm not sure.
>
> DR. BROOKS: Gee, you really know a lot about grasshoppers, so I'm wondering: How would a grasshopper let her trainer know

if the trainer was pushing too hard? [I wanted to introduce the notion that Meredith could assume some responsibility and ownership for offering feedback; as we have noted, a sense of ownership is an important feature of resilience.]

MEREDITH: The grasshopper just wouldn't jump [an oppositional way of coping].

DR. BROOKS: Anything else?

MEREDITH: The grasshopper could jump in the wrong direction [another oppositional way of coping].

DR. BROOKS: Would the trainer know why the grasshopper wasn't jumping or was jumping in the wrong direction? [As in a previous comment, I wanted to reinforce Meredith's responsibility for what transpired in therapy. I also wanted to encourage Meredith to communicate her feelings.]

MEREDITH: No.

DR. BROOKS: Hmm. That's a problem. If a trainer really wanted to help and was pushing too hard but didn't know it, he couldn't be helpful, and the grasshopper couldn't learn. [In part, I was attempting to highlight the self-defeating nature of the grasshopper's coping strategies, and to communicate that the trainer could be of help.]

MEREDITH: Yeah.

DR. BROOKS: That's a problem that needs solving. [An important message to communicate is that problems can be solved—certainly a significant component of resilience.]

MEREDITH: Yeah.

We return to therapy with Meredith and the use of storytelling later in this chapter.

Clinical Case Example: Don't Feed the Wolf Trash!

Jim, a 9-year-old boy, was referred for poor school performance, low self-esteem, and impulsivity. During the first session, he moved quickly around the office and eventually selected a wolf puppet to place on his hand. As the wolf, he uttered, "I only want good food in here and not trash." He also talked about a boy and a dog who went too fast and the dog was killed by a car. Interestingly, Jim had an uncle whose poodle had recently run into the street and had been hit by a truck and killed.

Jim then returned to the wolf puppet and repeated its desire for good food. The following dialogue ensued:

> DR. BROOKS: (*Talking to the wolf*) Do you think I would give you trash?
>
> JIM: (*As the wolf*) Maybe.
>
> DR. BROOKS: Has anyone ever given you trash? [I wanted to determine the possible basis of his statement or concern.]
>
> JIM: I can't remember.
>
> DR. BROOKS: Do you know why I would want to give you good food? [I was interested in Jim's perception of why he was coming to therapy.]
>
> JIM: No.
>
> DR. BROOKS: Any ideas at all?
>
> JIM: I'm not sure.
>
> DR. BROOKS: (*Still talking with the wolf*) Well, can I tell you?
>
> JIM: OK.
>
> DR. BROOKS: I'd like to give you good food, so that you can grow and learn to do things better and feel better. [With this statement, I began to introduce the goals of therapy.] But do you know what?
>
> JIM: No, what?
>
> DR. BROOKS: If you sometimes feel you don't like the food in here, I really want you to tell me, so that I can find the best food to help you grow. [I was trying to reinforce the notion that I welcomed Jim's playing an active role in the relationship, including providing feedback.]
>
> JIM: OK.

In this interaction, involving Jim as a wolf who was hungry and wanted to make certain only good food was offered, my main goals were both to introduce the notion that I was someone who could help Jim to grow, and, as importantly, to emphasize that Jim's input and involvement were necessary features of their interaction. Brooks and Goldstein (2004) emphasize the significance of what they call "personal control," or taking ownership and responsibility for one's experiences, as an essential feature of resilience throughout the lifespan. The wolf character appeared in many of Jim's therapy sessions, facilitating my interactions with him and helping him to cope more effectively with the problems he faced.

STORYTELLING AND THE CREATIVE CHARACTERS TECHNIQUE

The information gathered about the child in the diagnostic evaluation and the first few sessions of treatment provides rich content for the ongoing use of storytelling in therapy to promote resilience. While many child clinicians have used storytelling, it was Gardner (1971, 1972, 1975) who popularized it through his Mutual Storytelling technique, as well as through such well-known therapeutic games as The Talking, Feeling, and Doing Game and The Storytelling Card Game. His books and games are now used by many child therapists.

Gardner would introduce a child to his Mutual Storytelling technique by saying, "Boys and girls, welcome to Dr. Gardner's Make-Up-A-Story Television Program." He would then invite the child to create a story guided by several parameters, including that the story contain elements of adventure, that it not be something the child had viewed on television or in the movies, and that it include a moral or lesson at the end. After each child patient completed a story, Gardner would use the same characters and settings to help the child create a story that highlighted more constructive ways of coping than was evident in the patient's original story. In essence, through the ongoing development of these stories, Gardner developed a vehicle through which to teach children about more adaptive strategies for expressing their thoughts and emotions.

I (Robert Brooks) found Gardner's storytelling technique intriguing and informative, and it led me to cultivate my own interest in the therapeutic power of stories. However, I began to modify Gardner's approach to accommodate my own style and to pursue goals that I perceived to be more beneficial with my child patients. I labeled my storytelling technique "Creative Characters" and drew heavily on the use of metaphors (Brooks, 1981, 1985, 1987), including those that emerged in the first few sessions with a child.

The Creative Characters technique involves the therapist's selecting major issues confronting the child. As we have noted above in discussing the first few sessions of therapy, these issues are often raised by children themselves. If a child does not initially offer metaphors (as Meredith did with the grasshopper or Jim with the wolf), the therapist may introduce such representations, based on initial knowledge of the child's issues. Once certain characters and the situations they face are identified, the therapist and child can elaborate on this content during subsequent sessions to address issues in the character's (child's) life.

There are several ways in which Creative Characters differs from the Mutual Storytelling technique. I have found that requesting a child to identify a moral or lesson from the story frequently seems forced and artificial because it does not always evolve naturally from the storyline. I have found that children can learn from the stories in the absence of a stated moral.

I have also discovered that the inclusion of certain characters within the story enhances the elaboration and impact of the story. One figure I introduce in all of the stories is a representation of myself as the therapist. This permits me to ask questions and have a dialogue within the story, rather than offering comments and asking questions as an observer outside the story. The presence of this therapist figure contributes to a noticeably richer, more natural dialogue than when this figure is not present.

The second figure that surfaces in many of the stories created in my sessions was actually first introduced by Jeremy, a 10-year-old patient. In his story, without any prompting, Jeremy assumed the role of an "investigative reporter," interviewing different people about an incident that had taken place. In real life, Jeremy had been accused of bullying several peers at school—an action he denied or minimized by saying, "I was only fooling around. Everyone fools around." Jeremy played both the reporter as well as other students "to get to the truth." He allowed me to join in as a second reporter, and I used this position as an opportunity to interview Jeremy and the other students; I sometimes assumed the role of the other students as well.

As the story evolved, I, as the reporter, helped Jeremy to understand different points of view and to appreciate that what he considered "only fooling around" was experienced by his peers as hurtful. One benefit of this perspective taking was to nurture Jeremy's capacity for empathy and problem solving—both dimensions of resilience.

In addition to the newscaster's or news reporter's being able to enter into a dialogue with the patient's characters, I have found that some patients derive another benefit from including this figure. Often, using an audio recorder, I will at the end of a story highlight several of the main points that have arisen during the story. At the start of the next session, the newscaster offers a brief summary of the previous session's key themes, which serves as a natural segue for continuing the discussion of these themes in the current session. I have found that many of my patients enjoy these "reviews" of the issues, often requesting to play the reporter. Particularly revealing are the occasions when a patient offers a summary that is noticeably different from my recollection of what transpired during the previous session. Such differences in perception elicit rich material for further discussion.

The Creative Characters technique provides an avenue to reinforce a basic skill associated with resilience: problem solving. It invites children through the different characters, especially the figure that most clearly represents the child, to think of the problem and different possible options for confronting the problem. It is not unusual for patients to take what they have learned from these different characters and apply it to situations in their own life without necessarily leaving the boundaries of the story. Jennifer, a 7-year-old girl who was very fearful, learned more effective ways of coping from Alice, the character who represented her in one of the stories she and I created. Jennifer told me that she often thought of what Alice would do if faced with the same challenges.

An additional benefit that accrues from storytelling techniques such as Creative Characters is a positive impact on cognitive functioning, which is intimately related to problem-solving skills. Therapists frequently see children who display such cognitive difficulties as distractibility, limited attention span, and poor memory. Such youngsters initially require extensive external support in therapy to assist them to focus and attend, so that they can develop the cognitive skills necessary to master their problems.

The Creative Characters technique can provide such support and strengthen cognitive processes in at least two major ways. First, since children typically find the format and characters that appear in the stories very interesting, they become increasingly motivated to focus on the stories, thereby slowly enhancing their ability to attend and sustain attention.

Second, the nature of the technique encourages the child (with the therapist's input) to delineate and then elaborate upon selected aspects of the personalities and behaviors of the different characters, permitting movement away from simplistic notions and solutions to a more thoughtful, realistic understanding of behaviors. This elaboration that transpires in the ongoing creation of the story promotes the child's capacity to focus on and understand his or her own feelings and thoughts in a more sophisticated, more integrated, and less fragmented manner. Thus Creative Characters storytelling embraces both cognitive and affective functioning, with each domain influencing the other.

Clinical Case Examples: The Creative Characters Technique in Child Therapy

As we have emphasized throughout this chapter, storytelling can be used to nurture a resilient mindset in our child patients, replacing doubt, despair, and pessimism with hope, optimism, and a sense of personal control. The following case examples illustrate the application of the Creative Characters technique to reinforce resilience. As we have done in the dialogues earlier in this chapter, we offer comments explaining the rationales for some of the interventions.

"I'm Afraid to Try"

Many children we see in therapy fear failure and the humiliation that frequently accompanies setbacks. To avoid the emotional pain and hurt of humiliation, children may resort to actions that prove self-defeating, including avoiding or quitting tasks that they believe may eventuate in failure. Timmy, age 9, had had a seizure disorder since the age of 4. On a few occasions, Timmy had fallen down while having a seizure and had lost consciousness. Perhaps the scariest moment came when he had a seizure while in a pool and was rescued by the lifeguard. Timmy was also beset with learning and attention problems that contributed to a high level of frustration in school. Timmy's parents and teacher observed that when he was asked to engage in a new task, he immediately displayed a knee-jerk reaction: shouting "No!" and exclaiming that the task was stupid.

In therapy Timmy said little and was not easy to engage. His play was unfocused and frenetic, taking the form of shooting darts wildly around the office or scribbling on a piece of paper and then tearing the paper in half. His attention seemed limited at best. I (Robert Brooks) decided to introduce Creative Characters with two main goals: (1) to help identify Timmy's fears so that they could be confronted, and (2) to help him to settle down and focus by attending to the story.

An opportunity arose for storytelling when Timmy offered a comment without prompting. He said that he had seen a circus on television and liked the elephant act. When I inquired what Timmy liked, the only thing he could recall was the elephants' walking around in a circle, each elephant balancing on its hind legs with the other legs on the back of the elephant in front of it. This image of balancing on two legs appeared to be especially meaningful, given Timmy's history of seizures and falling down. I encouraged Timmy to tell me more about elephants, but Timmy declined to do so. I decided to take the initiative, informing Timmy that I knew a great story about elephants. Timmy looked surprised and asked, "What kind of story?" Timmy's interest suggested that the door was open, even slightly, for me to begin creating a story that might represent key issues in Timmy's life.

I proceeded to tell Timmy that there was once an elephant named "Johnny Scared," who wanted to perform an act in the circus that would require Johnny to learn to walk on two feet with the other elephants. (I will sometimes call a character by a certain name to capture a major emotion that can be used throughout the story—a name that is open to modification as the story progresses. Also, since Timmy had been intrigued by the image of elephants walking on two feet, it seemed a good fit to have the main figure of the story learn to walk on two feet.)

I, as Johnny Scared, voiced that he wanted to learn to walk on two feet, but he didn't know if he could. I acted out the role, straining to walk on two feet but constantly falling over. The physical acting out of stories often enhances fantasy production and the elaboration of the main themes. Saltz and his colleagues (e.g., Saltz, Dixon, & Johnson, 1977) found that the addition of physical enactment of fantasy themes for young children promoted cognitive development, impulse regulation, and fantasy production. Sensory–motor or action experiences appear to lay the foundation for later cognitive development (Brooks, 1981; Gaskill & Perry, 2014).

Timmy looked amused as I made believe I was trying to walk on two feet and kept falling over (a behavior that in many ways paralleled Timmy's losing consciousness and falling when he had a seizure). Timmy's interest was piqued when I kept moaning, "I can't take it anymore, and I'm going to quit. I'll never learn to stand on my own two feet. It's too hard to do this." When I assumed this stance of quitting, Timmy eventually demonstrated a behavior that we have seen with other children: They take on the role of the encouraging therapist. Timmy said, "You can learn to walk." At this point, I said that I needed someone to train me, and I asked Timmy to be the "animal trainer" (the therapist role).

Timmy assumed this role with enthusiasm, almost as if feelings of hope, which had been dormant, were now encouraged to come forth. He gave me directions about how to walk on two feet, although I at first played the "resistant" patient, moaning and groaning and verbalizing the fears that Timmy harbored.

In subsequent sessions, Timmy played the role of Johnny while I became the animal trainer. To facilitate the flow of the story, I introduced the character of a newspaperman who was assigned to write a story about the circus and Johnny Scared. In one session, I as Johnny Scared told the reporter how I had never been able to do things very well and I just wanted to quit, but that when I did quit the other elephants teased me, which made me feel even worse.

Interestingly, as Johnny Scared was slowly learning to walk on two feet, Timmy's teacher reported a noticeable decrease in his avoidant behavior at school and his willingness to accept her help. Also, in the sessions with me, Timmy made a sign for Johnny Scared that read, "Don't quit." His teacher reported that he had written the same words in his notebook at school. Very significantly and very poignantly, during one of the final weeks of the story, Timmy announced that Johnny Scared needed a new name. I inquired of Timmy, "What do you think should be the new name?"

Timmy's response vividly captured the power of metaphors. Without hesitation, he replied, "Johnny Brave." In the next few weeks, I helped Timmy to describe the differences between Johnny Scared and Johnny Brave, with a major focus on finding more adaptive ways of coping when faced with challenges. As sometimes occurs in therapy, Timmy himself drew comparisons between his real life and the story; he would speak about how he was becoming less scared and more brave in school and at home.

"Why Aren't You Living Together?"

Lisa, age 6, was referred to me (Robert Brooks) following her parents' separation and the brief hospitalization of her mother for depression and an overdose of sleeping pills. Initially, Lisa was very stressed and did not want to talk about what had happened. She became agitated at any mention of the family situation, frequently running out of the office. Lisa's teacher reported that she was having trouble attending to tasks in class, and that she would alternate between being sullen and withdrawn on the one hand and suddenly yelling at classmates on the other.

Lisa's mother thought that Lisa felt some responsibility for the parents' separation and for the mother's becoming depressed and having to be hospitalized. Lisa had told both of her parents that in the future she would be a "good girl and not a bad girl," suggesting that she perceived her behavior as contributing to the current situation in the family. In addition, the mother reported a theme that is not unusual among children whose parents have separated: "I think Lisa feels responsible for bringing her father and me back together, and also for making me feel happy." Lisa indeed was carrying a heavy burden, especially for one so young and vulnerable. It was not surprising how scared and agitated she was.

Given how quickly Lisa became overwhelmed, and how difficult it was for her to express her emotions and thoughts in a more constructive manner, I decided to introduce a story. My goal was to use storytelling as a means to capture Lisa's family situation; to help her share her feelings and thoughts in a more focused and less frightening way; to correct distortions she held about her responsibility in causing and remedying the family turmoil; and to help her discover effective ways of coping with her sadness and anger.

Since Lisa was quick to tell me to be quiet and then to run out of my office, I decided that I had to present the story in a way that would short-circuit this usual response and allow her to listen to the story without fleeing the scene. I felt that to do so, I would need to create a situation that permitted Lisa some sense of control, encouraged her input, and engaged her problem-solving capabilities—all features of a resilient mindset.

In considering the characters that should inhabit the story, I asked both parents about some of Lisa's interests. Both noted that she loved chicks, especially after she visited a farm that had chickens. Given this information, I decided that the story would revolve around a little chicken.

Prior to one of my sessions with Lisa, I drew a picture of a little chick that I called "Chicky Worried," who was talking to a dog named "Dr. Sam." (Although I contemplated having Lisa name the chick, I decided that given the way in which I planned to introduce the story, it would be easiest if I gave the chick a name. I also felt that if Lisa wanted to do so, she could change the chick's name and/or create one or two other chicks with different names.) I put the picture of the chick and dog on the wall in my office, where Lisa could not miss seeing it. I also recorded the beginning of a story about Chicky Worried. When she entered the office, Lisa immediately noticed the picture and asked, "What's that?"

I told Lisa that I liked to make up stories about animals, and I also liked children to add to or change my stories to make them more interesting. I added,

> "I like to draw pictures for the story, and this one (*pointing to the one hanging on the wall*) is about a little chick named Chicky Worried and a dog named Dr. Sam. I recorded the beginning of a story about Chicky Worried. I would like to play it for you, since I could really use your help in telling me what you think about the story, what else should be in the story, and whether other kids would be interested in it."

I intentionally used the word "help," since an integral feature of a resilient mindset is the belief that one is making a positive difference in the world and helping others. We feel that such a belief also provides children with a sense of purpose and personal control, and of being proactive rather than reactive—other components of resilience.

My invitation to Lisa, a gesture she was not expecting, helped to distract her from her typical responses of telling me to be quiet and running from my office. She told me that she would listen to the story. I noticed that as I was starting the recording, Lisa displayed more eye contact and was more focused than in previous sessions.

The story involved a rooster and hen (representing Lisa's parents) who loved each other, got married, and had a beautiful little chick they named Chicky. However, after a few years the rooster and hen began to fight, and one day they told Chicky that they were not happy together and the rooster was moving to live on a nearby farm. The rooster and hen both told Chicky how much they loved her, and the rooster assured her that he would see her often.

Chicky asked her parents to stay together, but they said it was not something they could do. Chicky pleaded that she would be a good chick if they didn't separate, but they told her she was a good chick and they were not separating because of her. The rooster moved to another farm, and while Chicky saw him often, she was sad. Making Chicky feel more upset was the fact that her mother cried a great deal. Chicky wanted to make her mother happy, but she wasn't able to do so.

The recorded story had only a few minutes left when Lisa inquired, "What did Chicky do?" I stopped the tape recorder and pointed to the picture I had drawn of Chicky and Dr. Sam and placed on the wall. I told Lisa that Dr. Sam was a dog who liked to help young animals feel less sad and mad, and that he began to talk with Chicky. Given Lisa's obvious interest in the story, I invited her to help create the rest of the story with me. She agreed to do so.

I was impressed by how quickly Lisa became involved in storytelling. It afforded her a safe medium through which to express her thoughts and emotions without becoming overwhelmed as she had in previous sessions.

Lisa continued the story with content that was not unexpected. She said that Chicky asked Dr. Sam to speak with her parents about getting back together, which Dr. Sam agreed to do. Lisa said, "Dr. Sam spoke to Chicky's mommy and daddy, and they got back together again and the daddy moved back home, and Chicky was happy."

Seemingly magical endings are not unusual when children assume the role of authors or coauthors of the Creative Characters stories. It is a challenge for therapists to help children use the story to accept the reality of situations they confront in their lives and to cope more effectively with these situations. Sensitivity and empathy on the therapists' part are essential in accomplishing this task, lest children feel that their voices are not being heard and that adults are dismissing their worries.

I complimented Lisa on her story, but then asked if I might create another story with Dr. Sam and Chicky Worried for us to consider. Lisa replied, "But I like my story." I replied, "I also like your story, but sometimes it's good to have a couple of different stories to talk about. So is it OK for me to tell mine, and if you have any questions about my story, please let me know?" Lisa said it was OK.

My story continued with the theme introduced by Lisa, from the point at which Chicky asked Dr. Sam to speak with her parents about getting back together. However, my story took a different course than that suggested by Lisa. In my version, to which Lisa listened attentively without interrupting, Dr. Sam said to Chicky that he would speak with her parents, but he didn't know if he could bring them back together. In fact, Dr. Sam reported to Chicky after speaking with her parents that they told him they would not be getting back together.

I continued to play the roles of both Dr. Sam and Chicky. As Chicky, I screamed, "Daddy has to move back with us!"

As Dr. Sam, I responded empathically, "I know you would like them to get together again, and I can see how upset you are. Any chicky would be. But your parents told me that your daddy won't be moving back home, but that he will see you a lot and they both love you."

Lisa told me she liked her story better. I replied that I was glad she told me which story she preferred, but what we could do was to keep both stories. Lisa hesitated, but then agreed with my suggestion. Interestingly, in subsequent sessions Lisa deferred to my story, in which I introduced additional messages, all guided by the goal of nurturing her resilience. For example, to reinforce the issue of personal control, Dr. Sam told Chicky that she was not responsible either for her parents' separating or for getting them back together. Although at first it was difficult for Chicky to accept Dr. Sam's opinion, eventually she was able to do so.

Relatedly, Dr. Sam told Chicky that he knew it was upsetting to see her mother sad, but that as much as she wanted her mother to feel better, it was not her responsibility as a little chick to make her mother happy. However, he told her that he had found another doctor like him to help her mother feel less sad, and that this other doctor was also speaking with Chicky's father (this paralleled what was occurring in real life).

Lisa became increasingly involved with the ongoing story during the following year of treatment. She assisted me in drawing pictures related to the themes of the story. One drawing portrayed Chicky visiting her father, and another depicted her mother speaking to her own doctor.

Since a significant component of a resilient mindset is the belief that one has a purpose in life and is making a contribution to the well-being of others, I asked Chicky if she would be willing to speak with another little chick whose parents were separating. Lisa immediately said yes. I invited Lisa to play Chicky while I played the role of the other chick. This provided a wonderful opportunity for me as the other chick to share with Chicky my feelings of sadness, anger, and worry (feelings similar to Lisa's when her parents separated), and for Lisa to respond in what amounted to the therapist's role.

One suggestion that Lisa made to the little chick was to speak with a doctor like Dr. Sam. As the little chick, I asked, "Why?" Lisa replied, "Dr. Sam really knows how I feel and was able to help me, and he also helped my parents."

A year after therapy ended, Lisa and her parents were all doing much better when a truly tragic event occurred: Lisa's father, who had not previously been ill, suddenly suffered a heart attack and died. Lisa's mother called to tell me this terrible news and said that Lisa wanted to come to see me. When Lisa entered my office, she looked very sad. Lisa and I spoke about how painful it was to lose her father. Lisa lamented, "I will never see him again."

I empathized with Lisa's sadness at the idea of never again seeing her father. We eventually spoke about the many memories that Lisa would continue to have of her father—memories that she would always carry with her. Although we talked very directly about her father's death, something occurred that bore testimony to the power of storytelling. Lisa asked me if we could continue with the story of Dr. Sam and Chicky. I said yes. Lisa asked me to play Dr. Sam, and she took the role of Chicky, informing him of her father's death. Lisa returned to a known, safe haven in which to express her emotions and thoughts.

For the next several months as part of each session, Lisa alternated between her real-life story and the story of Chicky. In fact, they were both one story, but she chose the medium through which she felt more comfortable at any given time. The story included her father's sudden death, his funeral, her sadness, and her increased capacity to deal with such a difficult loss. When we were engaged in the Chicky story, she and I drew several pictures—including one of Chicky visiting her father's gravesite, and another of Chicky looking at photos that included her with her father as a way of holding onto memories of their times together.

I saw Lisa for several more months and was impressed with both her and her mother's increasing resilience. When we finished this second round of therapy, I let Lisa know that I was available to speak with her at any time. Lisa's mother called me every 3–4 months. I did not have any additional sessions with Lisa, given how well she was doing. The characters of Chicky and Dr. Sam had provided Lisa a safe means by which to manage a very difficult situation in her life.

Back to Meredith and the Grasshopper

Earlier in this chapter, we described the initial sessions with Meredith and her introduction of the metaphor of the grasshopper. Given Meredith's interest in the dialogue that ensued, I (Robert Brooks) then introduced the Creative Characters technique, informing Meredith that I was also interested in grasshoppers and would love to create a story about them with her. Meredith eagerly agreed and actively participated in the development of the story.

The story involved a girl grasshopper who had difficulty jumping, which made her feel insecure in comparison with other grasshoppers. Meredith also added that the grasshopper felt she was being pushed too hard by her parents and teacher. In the story, she reluctantly went to see a grasshopper trainer, who conveyed several important messages: (1) He wanted to help the grasshopper learn to jump far and straight, but the grasshopper should let him know if he pushed on her too hard; (2) although he could help, the grasshopper would have to play an important role in the training program; (3) continuing to refuse to jump and/or to jump in the wrong direction might once have served the grasshopper as useful strategies, but at the present time they were not very helpful; and (4) he could also speak with the grasshopper's parents and teacher, so that they would learn not to push too hard, but instead become more supportive (this last point was accomplished, in part, through regularly scheduled meetings with Meredith's parents and her teacher).

Meredith enjoyed being an active participant in the creation of the story, and for the most part she stayed within the metaphor and story throughout therapy. As noted earlier, it is not always necessary to venture into a patient's real world if the metaphors and stories of the therapy session are used by the patient outside the clinician's office (e.g., Ekstein, 1966; Haley, 1973). Most reassuring was that the grasshopper's progress in learning to jump straight and far was paralleled by a noticeable lessening of Meredith's oppositional behavior and temper tantrums.

CONCLUDING COMMENTS

We have been impressed by the enthusiasm and interest displayed by our child patients when metaphors and stories become a significant part of the therapeutic process. We believe that this enthusiasm is rooted in part in the experiences of developing a sense of mastery and competence, and thus of becoming increasingly resilient. Many of our child patients enter therapy burdened by feelings of helplessness and inadequacy; they are convinced that they have little if any ability to make things better or to determine what transpires in their lives.

Storytelling (such as the Creative Characters technique), and the metaphors embedded in these stories, allow children to adopt a more active role in solving their problems—one in which they become significant participants. This offers them hope against the prevailing attitude of defeatism. The stories constitute a safe vehicle through which they can move back and forth from the role of the therapist to the characters representing themselves. In this process, they can be the helper as well as the ones being helped; they can learn to observe and understand feelings and thoughts; and they can test solutions in therapy that can then be applied outside the therapist's office. As they help to create these stories, they can learn that they are "authors of their own lives," moving from a mindset filled with doubt and pessimism to one dominated by a resilient outlook.

We believe that these observations about the impact of metaphors and storytelling were captured in Timmy's pronouncement that the elephant Johnny Scared had a new name, Johnny Brave. The change in names represented a new metaphor that now guided Timmy's life—one filled with courage and perseverance. This shift in perspective and behavior, which was facilitated by the therapeutic use of storytelling, is one we would hope to witness in all of our child patients.

REFERENCES

Barker, P. (1985). *Using metaphors in psychotherapy.* New York: Brunner/Mazel.
Berg-Cross, G., & Berg-Cross, L. (1976). Bibliotherapy for young children. *Journal of Clinical Child Psychology, 5,* 35–38.
Brooks, R. (1981). Creative Characters: A technique in child therapy. *Psychotherapy, 18,* 131–139.

Brooks, R. (1983). Projective techniques in personality assessment. In M. D. Levine, W. B. Carey, A. C. Crocker, & R. Gross (Eds.), *Developmental-behavioral pediatrics* (pp. 974–989). Philadelphia: Saunders.

Brooks, R. (1984). Success and failure in middle childhood: An interactionist perspective. In M. D. Levine & P. Satz (Eds.), *Middle childhood: Development and dysfunction* (pp. 87–128). Baltimore: University Park Press.

Brooks, R. (1985). The beginning sessions of therapy: Of messages and metaphors. *Psychotherapy, 22,* 761–769.

Brooks, R. (1987). Storytelling and the therapeutic process for children with learning disabilities. *Journal of Learning Disabilities, 20,* 546–550.

Brooks, R. (2010). Power of mindsets: A personal journey to nurture dignity, hope, and resilience in children. In D. A. Crenshaw (Ed.), *Reverence in healing: Honoring strengths without trivializing suffering* (pp. 19–40). Lanham, MD: Jason Aronson.

Brooks, R., & Brooks, S. (2014). Creating resilient mindsets in children and adolescents: A strength-based approach for clinical and nonclinical populations. In S. Prince-Embury & D. H. Saklofske (Eds.), *Resilience interventions for youth in diverse populations* (pp. 59–82). New York: Springer.

Brooks, R., & Goldstein, S. (2001). *Raising resilient children.* New York: McGraw-Hill.

Brooks, R., & Goldstein, S. (2004). *The power of resilience.* New York: McGraw-Hill.

Brooks, R., & Goldstein, S. (2007). *Raising a self-disciplined child.* New York: McGraw-Hill.

Brooks, R., & Goldstein, S. (2011). The power of mindsets: Raising resilient children. In G. Koocher & A. La Greca (Eds.), *The parents' guide to psychological first aid: Helping children and adolescents cope with predictable life crises* (pp. 142–150). New York: Oxford University Press.

Crenshaw, D. A. (2006). *Evocative strategies in child and adolescent psychotherapy.* Lanham, MD: Jason Aronson.

Crenshaw, D. A. (Ed.). (2008a). *Child and adolescent psychotherapy: Wounded spirits and healing paths.* Lanham, MD: Jason Aronson.

Crenshaw, D. A. (2008b). *Therapeutic engagement of children and adolescents: Play, symbol, drawing, and storytelling strategies.* Lanham, MD: Aronson.

Crenshaw, D. A. (Ed.). (2010). *Reverence in healing: Honoring strengths without trivializing suffering.* Lanham, MD: Jason Aronson.

Dolan, Y. M. (1985). *A path with a heart: Ericksonian utilization with resistant and chronic clients.* New York: Brunner/Mazel.

Drewes, A. A. (2014). Helping foster care children heal from broken attachments. In C. A. Malchiodi & D. A. Crenshaw (Eds.), *Creative arts and play therapy for attachment problems* (pp. 197–214). New York: Guilford Press.

Ekstein, R. (1966). *Children of time and space, of action and impulse.* New York: Appleton-Century-Crofts.

Erickson, M. H., & Rossi, E. L. (1979). *Hypnotherapy: An exploratory casebook.* New York: Irvington.

Frey, D. E. (1993). Learning by metaphor. In C. E. Schaefer (Ed.), *The therapeutic powers of play* (pp. 223–239). Northvale, NJ: Jason Aronson.

Gardner, R. A. (1971). *Psychotherapeutic communication with children: The Mutual Storytelling technique.* New York: Science House.

Gardner, R. A. (1972). *Dr. Gardner's stories about the real world.* Englewood Cliffs, NJ: Prentice-Hall.

Gardner, R. A. (1975). *Psychotherapeutic approaches to the resistant child.* New York: Jason Aronson.

Gardner, R. A. (1993). Mutual Storytelling. In C. E. Schaefer & D. M. Cangelosi (Eds.), *Play therapy techniques* (pp. 199–209). Northvale, NJ: Jason Aronson.

Gaskill, R. L., & Perry, B. D. (2014). The neurobiological power of play: Using the Neurosequential Model of Therapeutics to guide play in the healing process. In C. A. Malchiodi & D. A. Crenshaw (Eds.), *Creative arts and play therapy for attachment problems* (pp. 178–196). New York: Guilford Press.

Gil, E. (2014). The creative use of metaphor in play and art therapy with attachment disorders. In C. A. Malchiodi & D. A. Crenshaw (Eds.), *Creative arts and play therapy for attachment problems* (pp. 52–66). New York: Guilford Press.

Goldings, H. J. (1974). Focus on feelings: Mental health books for the modern world. *Journal of Child Psychiatry, 13,* 374–377.

Gordon, D. (1978). *Therapeutic metaphors.* Cupertino, CA: Meta.

Haley, J. (1973). *Uncommon therapy: The psychiatric techniques of Milton H. Erickson.* New York: Norton.

Keith, C. R. (1968). The therapeutic alliance in child psychotherapy. *Journal of the American Academy of Child Psychiatry, 7,* 31–43.

Kopp, R. R. (1995). *Metaphor therapy: Using client-centered metaphors in psychotherapy.* New York: Brunner/Mazel.

Kopp, S. (1971). *Guru: Metaphors from a psychotherapist.* Palo Alto, CA: Science & Behavior Books.

Korchin, S. J. (1976). *Modern clinical psychology.* New York: Basic Books.

Lankton, C. H., & Lankton, S. R. (1989). *Tales of enchantment: Goal-directed metaphors for adults and children in therapy.* New York: Brunner/Mazel.

Malchiodi, C. A., & Crenshaw, D. A. (Eds.). (2014). *Creative arts and play therapy for attachment problems.* New York: Guilford Press.

Mills, J. C., & Crowley, R. J. (1986). *Therapeutic metaphors for children and the child within.* New York: Brunner/Mazel.

Mills, J. C., & Crowley, R. J. (2014). *Therapeutic metaphors for children and the child within* (2nd ed.). New York: Routledge.

Nickerson, E. (1975). Bibliotherapy: A therapeutic medium for helping children. *Psychotherapy: Theory, Research, and Practice, 12,* 258–261.

Robertson, M., & Barford, F. (1970). Story-making in psychotherapy with a chronically ill child. *Psychotherapy: Theory, Research, and Practice, 7,* 104–107.

Saltz, E., Dixon, D., & Johnson, J. (1977). Training disadvantaged preschoolers on various fantasy activities: Effects on cognitive functioning and impulse control. *Child Development, 48,* 367–380.

Schaefer, C. E., & Cangelosi, D. M. (Eds.). (1993). *Play therapy techniques.* Northvale, NJ: Jason Aronson.

Schaefer, C. E., & Drewes, A. A. (Eds.). (2014). *The therapeutic powers of play: 20 core agents of change* (2nd ed.). Hoboken, NJ: Wiley.

Segal, J. (1988). Teachers have enormous power in affecting a child's self-esteem. *Brown University Child Behavior and Development Newsletter, 10,* 1–3.

Seymour, J. W. (2010). Resiliency-based approaches and the healing process in play therapy. In D. A. Crenshaw (Ed.), *Reverence in healing: Honoring strengths without trivializing suffering* (pp. 71–84). Lanham, MD: Jason Aronson.

Seymour, J. W. (2014). Resiliency as a therapeutic power of play. In C. E. Schaefer & A. A. Drewes (Eds.), *The therapeutic powers of play: 20 core agents of change* (2nd ed., pp. 241–263). Hoboken, NJ: Wiley.

Seymour, J. W., & Erdman, P. E. (1996). Family play therapy using a resiliency model. *International Journal of Play Therapy, 5,* 19–30.

Shure, M. B. (1996). *Raising a thinking child.* New York: Pocket Books.

Shure, M. B., & Aberson, B. (2013). Enhancing the process of resilience through effective thinking. In S. Goldstein & R. Brooks (Eds.), *Handbook of resilience in children* (2nd ed., pp. 459–480). New York: Springer.

Weiner, B. (1974). *Achievement motivation and attribution theory.* Morristown, NJ: General Learning Press.

White, M., & Epston, D. (1990). *Narrative means to therapeutic ends.* New York: Norton.

Zeig, J. (1980). *A teaching seminar with Milton H. Erickson.* New York: Brunner/Mazel.

Chapter 4

"Dear Mr. Leprechaun"

Nurturing Resilience in Children
Facing Loss and Grief

DAVID A. CRENSHAW
JILLIAN E. KELLY

A child who suffered early parental bereavement; disruptions of early attachments; considerable bullying and taunting from peers in elementary and middle school, along with symptoms of depression; and, in those dark moods, occasional suicidal thoughts might not be expected to be a good student, a talented dancer, and a poet. But Nick (a fictitious name) was exactly that and at age 14 wrote the following poem:

> Fear is the pain inside of me
> Trapping these emotions I'm trying to free
> Changing this person I'm trying to be
> Sometimes I just want to flee
> I'm searching for an answer
> A cure to this cancer
> But as long as I keep trying
> I'm saving myself from dying

I (David A. Crenshaw) dare say that no mental health professional has ever been so articulate in describing the struggle with the dark moods of depression, which often feel as if they will never end. Nick's academic accomplishments (earned through persistent, hard work in order to overcome learning struggles associated with attention-deficit/hyperactivity disorder [ADHD], inattentive type); his talents as a dancer and a poet;

and his being an unusually kind and polite young person speak volumes about what it means to be resilient. Nick's kind heart touched me deeply when, prior to Christmas the year he was 12, he told me about a woman in his church whose saved-up money to buy Christmas presents for her family was stolen from her. Nick gave her a gift card and a $50 bill that he had received as an early Christmas present to help her buy gifts for her children. What enabled Nick to be so resilient? The answer is complex and includes many factors, but two that stand out are Nick's own determination and the consistent, loving support of his mother and adoptive father.

On a hot summer day, I (David A. Crenshaw) am sitting in a gazebo on the campus of the Children's Home of Poughkeepsie (CHP), talking with a 15-year-old Latina who I quickly realize has confronted more hardship, abuse (both physical and sexual), and trauma than most citizens in the United States will face in a typical lifetime. She is 3 days into her latest out-of-home placement, her third in the last 5 months. She will find out when she goes to court next month what her next placement will be. At the moment, this spirited and determined youth is in our Group Emergency Foster Care program while awaiting the court's decision about her next step. I will call her Kara. She is pleasant, smiles a lot, and we immediately find a common ground in our love for dogs. She has a dearly loved Springer Spaniel named Toby at her birth parents' home, and I work with a Facility Dog named Ace, a Golden Retriever that all the children and youth at CHP adore. Ace is not working today because of a brief illness. We talk, laugh, and share stories about our dogs. I've only spent a few minutes with Kara, but I am moved by her warm and engaging manner, and I find myself thinking that this is a person it would be hard not to like. Likeability is a factor that contributes greatly to resilience.

I look around, and sitting at picnic tables, on a bench swing, and on the ground are other adolescents whose lives have also been marked by repeated exposure to violence, abuse, trauma, poverty, and frequent disruption of attachments. They are all in out-of-home placements, and for most of them (as for Kara), this is not the first stop in their journey through foster care placements. On the faces of the other adolescents, their stories are clearly written. Except for Kara, I don't see a smiling face, laughter, or engaging and animated conversation. In fact, what I see are faces indicating to the world that their hearts, hopes, and dreams have been crushed too many times. There is a hardness, sometimes a bitterness, in their faces that clearly shows the mistrust intended to protect them from further unbearable hurt. Their faces do not beckon me to come closer. When I finish talking with Kara, and I approach the others, I do so slowly and cautiously. I make a friendly, welcoming bid that is in most cases acknowledged, but in a reserved, distant way. Since I've worked with such extremely hurting youth for more than four and a half decades now, I would not expect anything else. I feel incredible sadness that youthful vitality and unbridled hope have been brutally preempted in these teens, at the point when most young people are just beginning the pursuit of their dreams.

Kara in her short life has witnessed violence both in her home and in her inner-city neighborhood. She has directly experienced the kind of cruelty that we would hope no child would ever experience. Kara has seen with her own eyes what no child should ever see. She has suffered a depth of pain that we would never want any child to feel. But when Kara smiles, her face lights up with a warmth that is contagious. Her smiles, her laughs, and her stories are shared in a wholehearted, sincere way. Kara still retains her hopes and dreams. She entertains the possibilities of being either a veterinarian, or a lawyer who specializes in family law and can help families and children who have been abused and maltreated because she knows all too well what that is like. Kara, like many youth, engages in fantasies of becoming very rich. But what she wants to do with all that fantasized money is to help the poor, especially the homeless who sleep out in the cold with only a thin blanket. She tells me that she wanted to bring blankets and food to a particular homeless man in the wintertime who slept in the street near her birth mother's apartment. Her wish to do this sparked a violent argument with her mother. Her mother, whom Kara perceives as a bitter, unforgiving woman (and who probably has an abundance of her own disappointments in life), insisted that "This is our food, our blankets, and I am not going to let you give anything away."

I am deeply touched by Kara even on this first meeting. I am moved by the generosity of a heart that has been shattered by the cruelty of adults in her life; she misses a home of her own, but still wants to help the homeless if ever she should have a lot of money. I am moved by her wanting to help others in small ways, as well as her hoping and dreaming for a future when she may be able to help others in a bigger way. I tell Kara that she reminds me of a girl, a homeless teen, on the streets of New York City who held up a cardboard sign that said "Broke but not broken!" Like this adolescent, Kara is broke but far from broken. Her spirit and her inner strength are truly remarkable. When I tell her this, tears flow freely down her cheeks, and she says simply, "Thank you." I reply, "Kara, thank *you* because in just the short time I've met with you, you have given me more than enough inspiration for a lifetime."

This chapter is about Nick, Kara, a child named Leila who is described later, and so many other children whose stories have inspired us. These are the children we meet in child psychotherapy who, with courage, determination, and perseverance, beat the odds, meet the challenges, and ultimately prevail over the adversity they encounter. This chapter is also about what we can learn from these inspiring children. None of them arrived at our offices wearing a Superman or Superwoman cape, but they are stellar examples of resilience at its best, and there is much that such youngsters can teach us in addition to inspiring us. They intrigue us and excite our imaginations, as well as touch our hearts. They are genuine children and adolescents who maintain a robust spirit with hopes and dreams like any other young person, in spite of the adversity they have faced and the many obstacles that still stand in the way of fulfilling their hopes. We can't work with such children without their touching something deep inside of us and making us feel blessed that we are here to listen to and honor their stories. We also share some of our ideas and play therapy interventions for supporting and furthering the resilience process in children whose adversity includes grief and loss, which can take many forms but which are unique to each child.

GRIEF IN CHILDHOOD

Children who experience the death or other departure of a parent, or separation from a parent, are faced not only with tangible losses (the parent, other family members, home, school, neighborhood, and sometimes culture if a child is relocated to another country) but with intangible losses (dreams, hopes, plans, unity, and togetherness). All these losses must be mourned in a way that is unique to children because grief in childhood is often different from adult grief (Crenshaw, 2002). Children typically need to grieve in a developmentally sequenced way (James, 1989). Unlike adults (who typically immerse themselves in an intense but temporary state of mourning), young children typically grieve a little at a time, in keeping with the cognitive and emotional resources they currently possess. As they get older and their development progresses, they are able to grieve further as additional understanding, emotional resources, and coping resources become available to them. For example, a 5-year-old child who experiences the death of a parent can only go so far in expressing grief. At age 9, this child understands death more fully from a cognitive standpoint and has more verbal and emotional capacity to give expression to the grief. In adolescence, as the understanding of death reaches an adult level (i.e., the youth develops a cognitive appreciation of the finality, irreversibility, and inevitability of death), this same person may be able to go still further in the grieving process.

Children take longer to grieve fully for an important loss because they are constrained in their earlier years by developmental limitations. But just like adults, they do grieve. Surviving family members can help them go as far as possible at any one stage of development. Some children (actually a minority because of children's adaptability) may need the assistance of trained mental health professionals in working through their grief—and for young children, play therapy is often where they begin the journey.

PLAY THERAPY WITH GRIEVING CHILDREN

Play therapy and expressive art therapies offer distinct advantages in work with children's grief and loss issues, especially in the case of traumatic grief (please note that from here on in this chapter, we use "children" to refer to both children and adolescents). Schaefer and Drewes (2013) have named over 20 healing properties of play, including building resilience. Brown (2009) studied murderers in Texas prisons and found that the absence of play in their childhood was as important as any other factor in predicting their crimes. Brown also studied abused children at risk for antisocial behavior and found that play diminished their predisposition for violence. Play therapy allows children to approach the painful parts of their stories at a pace that they regulate, and at the safe distance provided by metaphor and symbolism. Symbolic play, posttraumatic play, metaphor, externalization, and miniaturization are specific aspects of play therapy that make it particularly safe and valuable to young children and adolescents in working through grief, and each of these components is now examined separately.

Symbolic Play

Children seek mastery through play when experiences or emotions are overwhelming. After a funeral of a loved one, for instance, children are frequently observed playing out with siblings or playmates their own version of a funeral, including a makeshift coffin and often a burial. This often occurs naturally in a child's home or neighborhood, without prompting or guidance on the part of a therapist. It is clear that these attempts at mastery are reflections of children's innate capacity for resilience, or what Ann Masten (2001, 2014) has called "ordinary magic." The same children may not be able to talk directly about their grief, but they can create symbolic representations in their play and actively attempt to assimilate their powerful feelings about, images of, and associations to such events. The symbolism may be disguised to the degree necessary to allow a child to engage safely in repeated attempts at mastery without getting overwhelmed or disrupted in the play. In play therapy, a therapist provides the props and the safe setting for a child to engage in such mastery play, but also serves as a trusted witness to the events and feelings that unfold. In addition, if the child gets stuck in attempts at mastery and repetitively enacts the adverse events without relief, then more active intervention by the therapist is called for because such repetition may be an indication of posttraumatic play.

Posttraumatic Play

The term "childhood traumatic grief" (CTG) was proposed by Cohen and Mannarino (2010; Mannarino & Cohen, 2011) to describe "a condition in which children whose loved ones die under traumatic circumstances develop trauma symptoms that impinge on the children's ability to progress through typical grief processes" (Mannarino & Cohen, 2011, p. 24). The critical exposure component in CTG protocols is gained in play scenarios or drawings or in sand play pictures, which provide sufficient symbolization to enable the child to keep the needed distance from the feelings that threaten to be overwhelming. When dealing with a devastating loss, for example, a child may repetitively play out with puppets a turtle looking for its mother. The turtle is sad. After these futile searches, the turtle is exhausted but won't give up looking. Another example might be an adolescent's drawing of his or her family that includes a sister who recently died, reflecting the youth's shock and current inability to fully acknowledge the loss. Each self-initiated exposure to a symbolic representation of the traumatic loss or grief allows graded and safe exposure, in keeping with the exposure component of CTG protocols. Since the child can break off the play at any moment, the child remains in control of the process, the timing, and the pacing. The child also determines the degree to which the symbolic representation is distant from the actual experience(s).

As Gil (Chapter 5, this volume) points out, posttraumatic play is also an indication of continuing attempts at mastery, stemming from the powerful drive to heal and recover from adversity that we call "resilience." Posttraumatic play, however, may require assistance on the part of the play therapist if the child is truly stuck. In that instance, repeated attempts at mastery through repetition of the symbolized adverse event(s) are not leading to relief from the anxiety and stress; the emotions may still be too overpowering to assimilate, and the child is feeling increasingly helpless and frustrated, in spite of these efforts and determination to gain mastery. The key features of posttraumatic play were originally described by Terr (1991), and Gil (1991) has described practical ways of intervening to advance the play toward the mastery the child is attempting to achieve. From an integrative framework, the play therapist moves toward a more directive approach and introduces new characters or new variations of the play scene, to empower the child to move forward and to become unstuck.

Metaphor

Metaphor is a symbolized form of condensed but precise communication (see Brooks & Brooks, Chapter 3, this volume, for a fuller discussion). As Gil (2014) has pointed out, "Our language is rich with metaphors that are used as a shorthand for other more complex concepts" (p. 160). When exhausted, we might say, for example, "My tank is running on empty." Joyce Mills and Richard Crowley (1986, 2014) have written eloquently about the use of therapeutic metaphors with children, and Mills is known for her work in applying the concepts of Milton Erickson (a pioneer in the use of metaphor) in play therapy. As Gil points out, play therapists as well as expressive arts therapists "have a profound recognition of the importance of clients' having the emotional distance and the inherent safety that they can enjoy as a result of having something stand in the place of something else. In addition, play and art therapists are taught to 'stay with' the metaphors created, rather than making jarring verbal interpretations of similarities between the metaphors and real life" (p. 159). Use of metaphor is another way that a child in play therapy can do grief work safely without becoming overwhelmed.

Externalization

When children externalize thoughts, feelings, and images that reside internally, something important happens in terms of mastery (Crenshaw, 2001b, 2006; Gil, 2010, 2014). Children externalize compelling facets of their inner world when they play out a drama with puppets, make a picture in a sand tray, draw or paint a picture, create a figure out of clay, or create a play scene in a family play house. What gets externalized is experienced as more manageable than that which remains internalized. Not only does it give the vague shapes and contours of the internal world a definition and clear form, but a child is able to stand back from it and assume a more objective view. Implicit in the externalization process is another potential powerful healing ingredient: sharing with a trusted adult who witnesses in a respectful and accepting way what the child has revealed.

Miniaturization

Play therapy and the expressive arts therapies also have in common the offering of opportunities to children to work with their "big problems" (which can be experienced as overwhelming) in a miniature, more manageable form (Gil, 2010). The very act of working with puppets or putting miniatures in the sand to make a picture, or drawing people or scenes, "shrinks" the problem to a more workable and manageable level for children—a level that enables them to gain mastery.

PLAY THERAPY INTERVENTIONS TO NURTURE RESILIENCE WITH GRIEVING CHILDREN

An examination of the therapeutic powers of play (Schaefer, 1993; Schaefer & Drewes, 2013), as eloquently explained by Seymour (2014; see also Chapter 2, this volume), makes it clear why one of these powers is resilience. The identified therapeutic mechanisms that enhance resilience include reducing anxiety and increasing problem solving; reducing self-blame; reducing blaming by others; reducing isolation and enhancing attachment; increasing self-esteem and self-efficacy; fostering creative problem solving; enhancing nurturing relationships beyond the playroom; and learning to make meaning of life's experiences (Seymour, 2014). In addition to these therapeutic mechanisms, each of the well-researched play therapy paths to resilience described in this section involves safe and respectful work with children and often their families, with emphasis on identifying and honoring strengths within each child and each family support system.

Modern attachment theory research has established clearly that one of the best buffers against adversity in life is secure attachment with parents or other primary caregivers (Gaskill & Perry, 2014; Schore, 2012; Siegel, 2012). The playful interactions that constitute the cornerstone of play therapy foster the attachment between child and therapist, and between the child and family members in such approaches as filial play therapy, family play therapy, and Theraplay. Those children who miss out on secure attachments early in life (and who are, in extreme cases, removed from their homes) can experience a reparative process in the secure attachment developed in therapy that once again is enhanced by playful interactions.

Child–Centered Play Therapy with Grieving Children

Child-centered play therapy (CCPT) explicitly honors the resilience of children, respects their innate healing resources, and pays tribute to their ability to pursue their own answers and solutions. Many times in CCPT, a play therapist simply stays out of the way and follows a child's lead, in keeping with the belief that children have the inner resources to find their own path to healing. CCPT is grounded in the writings of Virginia Axline (1969/1981, 1964/1986) and Garry Landreth (1982, 2012), and in the humanistic psychology of Clark Moustakas (1953, 1959, 1997). The theoretical basis of CCPT is Rogers's person-centered theory (1957, 1980; Rogers & Truax, 1976).

Daniel Siegel (2012) has discussed the valuable concept of "windows of tolerance":

> Each of us has a "window of tolerance" in which various intensities of emotional arousal can be processed without disrupting the functioning of the system. For some people, high degrees of intensity feel comfortable and allow them to think, behave, and feel with balance and effectiveness. For others, certain emotions (such as anger or sadness), or all emotions, may be quite disruptive to functioning even if they are active in even mild degrees. (p. 281)

CCPT is the treatment of choice for titrating the exposure to each individual child's window of tolerance for painful feelings of sadness, longing, guilt, fear, anger, and other typical emotions of grief because the child is deciding on the toys and themes to explore in a specific session and even at a specific point of time within the session.

Integrative Play Therapy with Grieving Children

While arguably CCPT is the safest and most respectful approach to gradual exposure to the painful events, memories, and feelings that permeate grief work, there are limitations that require astute and sensitive attunement on the part of the play therapist. As Siegel (2012) has explained, "The intensity of a specific emotional state may involve arousal and appraisal mechanisms outside awareness" (p. 281). Since unconscious factors play a role in the arousal intensity and the appraisal of meaning, a child may inadvertently exceed the boundaries of his/her window of tolerance, leading to disruption of functioning. To keep therapy safe, particularly in the case of traumatic grief, the graded exposure to the painful emotions and events accompanying grief calls for empathic attunement. The empathically attuned therapist will intervene when the child is unwittingly entering emotional territory that threatens to be overwhelming due to the unconscious factors identified by Siegel.

Adding to the challenges faced by the child and therapist is the importance of contextual factors. Siegel (2012) elaborates: "The width of a given individual's window of tolerance may vary, depending on the state of mind at a given time, the particular emotional valence, and the social context in which the emotion is being generated" (p. 282). The child's emotional state can vary significantly even within the same session. The strength of the therapeutic alliance will be another important variable to consider, as well as whether family members are present in the session and the degree to which the child experiences those family relationships as supportive.

A number of play therapists, who value the compelling advantages of CCPT in honoring children's strengths and innate capacity for healing, nevertheless utilize more directive approaches when children find it too painful to initiate discussion or to approach painful material even through symbolized play or expressive arts (Gil, 2006, 2010; James, 1989, 1994). An integrative play therapy approach uses both directive and nondirective (child-centered) methods, depending on the needs of the child (Drewes, 2011a, 2011b; Drewes, Bratton, & Schaefer, 2011; Goodyear-Brown, 2010; Seymour, 2014; Shelby, 2010; Shelby & Felix, 2005; Steele & Malchiodi, 2012; Webb, 2007, 2010). Of course, when the interventions are directed by the play therapist in contrast to CCPT, the therapist assumes greater responsibility for regulating the pace and intensity of the exposure to the painful events and emotions of grief, in sensitive attunement to the child's window of tolerance of the child at any particular moment in therapy.

Neurobiologically Informed Play Therapy with Grieving Children

An approach to grief informed by research in interpersonal neurobiology was first proposed by Crenshaw (2006). This approach includes a 12-stage treatment model for CTG, expanded from Crenshaw's (1990) original seven-step treatment for grief. Seymour (2014) has elaborated on the approach: "The model moves from an initial stage of establishing safety, through steps of grieving, to finding meaning and a coherent narrative to understand the traumatic loss" (p. 265).

Neuroscientific research on work with grieving children has continued to develop with Gaskill and Perry's (2014) Neurosequential Model of Therapeutics (NMT). The NMT offers play therapists working with grief a guide to sequencing interventions in keeping with a brain-mapping strategy. That is, it enables a therapist to select interventions according to the lowest part of the brain dysregulated at any given point in the therapy. The NMT interventions follow the sequence of brain development, beginning with the lower brain (brainstem, diencephalon, and cerebellum—the arousal level), then the midbrain (limbic brain—the emotional/relational level), and finally the higher brain (cortex—the level of thought, cognitions, reasoning). When therapists are working with children in highly dysregulated emotional states, Gaskill and Perry emphasize the need to calm and soothe the lower brain before emotional and cognitive interventions can be effective. This model is extremely valuable to play therapists working with the intense emotions of grief, particularly traumatic grief in children. The NMT can help a play therapist remain safely within a child's window of tolerance.

RESEARCH ON RESILIENCE DURING CHILDHOOD

The term "resilience" most commonly refers to relatively positive psychological outcomes in spite of exposure to severe adverse experiences (Rutter, 2006; Wolin & Wolin, 1992, 1993, 1996). Brooks and Goldstein (2001, 2003; see also Chapter 1, this volume) first introduced the concept of a "resilient mindset" that can be developed in all youth. In a recent publication, they explained: "The belief then is that every child capable of developing a resilient mindset will be able to deal more effectively with stress and pressure, to cope with everyday challenges, to bounce back from disappointments, adversity, and trauma, to develop clear and realistic goals, to solve problems, to relate comfortably with others, and to treat oneself and others with respect" (Goldstein & Brooks, 2013, p. 3).

Secure attachments in early life may be the best immunity available to individuals in the face of adversity (Gaskill & Perry, 2014). Research on resilience in young people faced with adversity has shown the importance of protective factors such as feeling loved by and connected to one's family, being well connected to peers, and having a good friendship group (Fuller, McGraw, & Goodyear, 2002). Children faced with a devastating loss such as the death of a parent develop more resilient outcomes when they are able to construct a coherent narrative of what happened and of its meaning for them (Balk, 1996; Lin, Sandler, Ayers, Wolchik, & Lauchen, 2004; Stokes, 2007). Positive emotional states also enhance resilience. Resilient people not only cultivate positive emotions in themselves to enhance coping, but tend to elicit positive emotions in others, which in turn facilitates a social context supportive of coping (Fredrickson, 2004). Bereavement is painful and difficult, but Bonanno (2009) emphasizes that it is a human experience like any other, and shares the view of Masten (2001, 2014) that people are typically resilient in the face of grief; however, there are many individual factors to consider.

Indeed, positive adjustment to adversity is complicated and depends on many variables, such as age (children are more vulnerable to adversity than adults); the duration of the adversity (a single trauma event vs. chronic exposure to adversity and/or multiple trauma events); intensity or severity of the trauma exposure (sometimes referred to as the "trauma dose gradient" in the literature); and the wide variation in response by individuals to the same trauma exposure—to name just a few of the factors to consider (Bonanno & Diminich, 2013; Goldstein & Brooks, 2013; Masten & Narayan, 2012; Rutter, 2006). There is a huge difference between recoveries from single-event trauma and from chronic adversity, although single-event trauma can cause long-term psychological problems if the trauma was severe or the exposed individual was vulnerable because of preexisting conditions. There is also a major difference between trauma exposures for children and for adults, as Gaskill and Perry (2014) have noted: "Although traumatic experiences can have a negative impact on adult functioning, the same adverse experiences have a much more deleterious impact on children because of the pervasive impact on development. Traumatic stress in adulthood affects a developed and functioning brain; trauma in childhood affects the organization and functioning of the developing brain" (p. 183). van der Kolk and his colleagues (2007) noted that adults suffering a traumatic event have been found to attain asymptomatic posttreatment status over time in 75% of cases, but that only 33% of children have been found to achieve this status over time. Yet we know that even in the case of unthinkable trauma and terror, children and families can rise above the adversity and live productive lives as adults (Crenshaw, 2013).

In sum, the research and writing of Bonanno (2009), Brooks and Goldstein (2001, 2003; Goldstein & Brooks, 2013), Masten (2001, 2014), and Rutter (2006) have well illustrated the amazing human capacity for resilience in the face of adversity. At the same time, many complexities must be considered (Bonanno & Diminich, 2013). Particularly in the case of children, who are still in the process of development, we must respect their innate resilience and malleability on the one hand, but also their greater vulnerability to adversity on the other. The recent work by Bonanno and Diminich (2013) has emphasized a wide range of trajectories following the death of a parent in childhood, with great attention to whether the traumatic loss is a single event or part of a cumulative pattern of loss and trauma. In the latter case, since a child's developmental process is compromised, the outcome is significantly negatively affected as a result of chronic stressors and repeated exposure to trauma. These findings make the case example presented below all the more remarkable: Leila faced with inspiring strength and resilience not one discrete encounter with adversity, but a wide range of challenges and setbacks related to her medical condition, along with cumulative stress as a result of this condition's effects on her functioning over the course of her development.

CLINICAL CASE EXAMPLE: LEILA

In July 2013 a beloved client, Leila, died in a tragic accident. I (Jillian E. Kelly) feel honored to share my reflections on this special person's resilience in the face of tangible and intangible losses, on the powerful therapeutic experience we co-created, and on a topic often left out of therapeutic publications—that is, the grieving process of the therapist. Leila was a joy to treat, and a treat to enjoy. She had a lot to say, and at the age of 10 she could comment on many topics with insight far beyond her years. She brought me a lot of understanding. Leila's story is both inspiring and vibrant, painful and tragic. It is my hope that this case presentation will highlight the importance of therapeutic presence (Crenshaw & Kenney-Noziska, 2014; Moustakas, 1997) in bringing about strength and resilience in both client and therapist, and that it will perhaps provide a renewed sense of purpose for those therapists who, like me, question their effectiveness from time to time.

There were countless moments during my initial years as a therapist when I thought about leaving the profession, having reviewed far too many devastating trauma histories, counted too many no-shows despite constant outreach, and tried desperately to comply with administrative demands. In the face of such challenges, therapists require a full stock of hope and purpose. My own stock consisted of the light of children's faces and the brightest light was Leila's. It was always her progress, and the delight I felt when working with her, that filled me with appreciation for my position and energy for our sessions on Friday afternoons. As a new and inexperienced therapist trying my hand at play therapy techniques and fumbling along the way, I learned from Leila the basics about how to interact with children—how to be really present beside them. Leila showed me how to appreciate the moment, and when I tried to take an intervention a step further than she was ready to go, she reminded me to "freaking slow down" and follow her lead. She was deliberate and direct in the most graceful of ways, and following her lead was incredibly rewarding.

Challenges, Obstacles, and Strengths in Leila during the Course of Therapy

Leila was diagnosed with chronic medical illnesses, including intractable epilepsy and right hemiparesis, during her childhood. She took over 15 pills per day, which produced side effects such as lethargy, bloating, and coarse hair growth. The illnesses themselves caused erratic twitching and shaking, cognitive deterioration, and considerable difficulty with fine motor skills such as holding a pencil. For several days each month, Leila and her parents would make their way to the hospital for inpatient procedures and monitoring. Other days she would return to the hospital's outpatient clinic for various scans and checkups. Leila disliked all this medical attention and the many procedures required of her. She was especially oppositional toward her mother and the medical staff, and fiercely defiant of the adjustments that had to be made.

Leila's problematic behaviors were the visible signs of the inner grief she was experiencing, having lost the ability to participate in the normal activities of childhood because of the need for ongoing medical appointments and procedures. Before her diagnosis, Leila's days had been full of exploration and adventure. A lover of nature and animals, she especially liked to visit the Museum of Natural History, collecting a pocket full of stones along her way home. When Leila's school principal suggested to her parents that they consider a transition to home schooling due to her medical illnesses, she was threatened with yet another loss—the loss of peer relationships and acceptance. An engaged and curious student, Leila enjoyed being part of the school community and was always eager to greet peers who were new, were shy, or otherwise needed a friend. I recall one session where Leila cried for 40 minutes. With the remaining 5 minutes we had in our session, I asked her what had happened that day to cause this steady stream of tears. Leila told me that she was crying for a classmate, a homeless child living in a shelter who was feeling particularly sad that day in school. Leila had a depth of empathy incredibly rare among even the most enlightened adults. It should be evident that Leila's school was fortunate to have such a caring student. Leila's mother advocated for her daughter, and, with accommodations, Leila was able to remain a member of her school community.

How Play Therapy Interventions Nurtured Resilience

Leila was initially referred by her mother for mental health treatment at our small community health center because of externalizing behaviors, such as becoming physically aggressive toward the adults in her life when she felt overwhelmed. To address these behaviors and the feelings that precipitated them, interventions included the following:

1. Engaging in directive and nondirective play therapy to foster Leila's confidence, control, and mastery within the therapeutic space.
2. Building upon Leila's feelings vocabulary, teaching affective identification, and helping her to label the specific feelings she experienced on a daily basis.
3. Offering guidance in the process of discovering natural coping skills, and teaching new coping skills.
4. Addressing the parents' needs by working as a team to infuse child-friendly fun into otherwise anxiety-producing medical visits.
5. Collaborating with school personnel to provide in-school supports and adjustments to expectations, with the purpose of ensuring that Leila would continue to feel accepted, confident, and valued as a unique member of the school community.
6. Partnering with members of the medical staff to exchange knowledge and advocate that they use the familiar metaphors of our sessions to change the tone of medical visits.

The treatment was designed by Leila as champion, myself as guide and container, and her mother as a skillfully creative parent participant. Our overarching goal for the treatment was to process the feelings Leila was experiencing related to the "unknowns" about her future health, and to address her intangible losses (of dreams, hopes, a normal childhood, and a sense of control within her body). Utilizing primarily play therapy techniques, the treatment would serve to invite Leila to reclaim her childhood.

Therapeutic Presence

I have read and conversed about the concept of "therapeutic presence" (Crenshaw & Kenney-Noziska, 2014; Moustakas, 1997), but it was not until I engaged in therapy with Leila that I really "got it." The frank feedback Leila gave me on the days I was actively listening, but especially on the days I was caught half-listening, brought me a lot of understanding. I also came to appreciate how good it felt when I removed the pressure to say the "right thing" and granted myself permission to simply enjoy the time with Leila and follow my instincts rather than a "one-stop-shopping" manual. We co-created our sessions on the basis of what unfolded naturally. Children are sensitive to social interactions, and their growth in relationships depends on the quality of the environment created (Blanco, Muro, & Stickley, 2014). I genuinely valued our time together, and this consistent display of positive regard became particularly important in working with Leila. As our therapeutic relationship developed, a natural flow followed. It was when Leila felt seen, heard, and related to in a way that was consistent with her own self-perception that she was free to integrate all of her experiences, leading to significant progress and resilience (Landreth, 2002).

Specific Interventions That Fostered Resilience

As part of the engagement process, I answered many of the questions Leila had for me. Being a woman of Irish heritage working in a predominantly Hispanic community, I was prepared for the inevitable curious cultural questions that children come up with. It became clear that for Leila, my being Irish meant that I was surely related to leprechauns, and my apparent affiliation with leprechauns quickly became far superior to any professional affiliation I might have. In traditional Irish folklore, the leprechaun is a symbol of luck. An industrious and mischievous little man, the leprechaun will only lead one to treasure if he is approached gently and steadily. It would appear that leprechauns and children have much in common!

Session after session, Leila would ask to hear stories of leprechaun life in Ireland; after gathering and examining her evidence, she ultimately decided that leprechauns were indeed real. We developed a technique, referred to as "Penpals," with the purpose of uncovering Leila's naturally creative internal resources and finding a medium to express her feelings from a safe distance (the distance between the city where we were working and County Galway is very, very great). Over several sessions, there was an exchange of letters between Leila and a certain leprechaun living on a carrot farm in County Galway. Here is Leila's first letter, reproduced with the permission of her mother:

Dear Mr. Leprechaun,
    I would love 800,000 pots of gold and a much better life without pills, twiching, or the hospital crap. Please help me get lots of luck

and never go back to the twiching or hospital or any of that junk.
Please please do all this for me and my freaking family. I also want
everything out of my stupid system and be normal.

    Love, Leila

In addition to the enjoyable anticipation this letter exchange provided, it gave Leila the opportunity to seek guidance and comfort, and
to express her grief. A compassionate child, she recognized the impact
of her illnesses on her family members and what they were missing out
on as a result of her illnesses. She was also aware of how she was seen
by her peers and deeply felt the loss of normality in body functioning.
"Disenfranchised grief" (Crenshaw, 2001b) is a grief that is fully experienced by the individual but not easily recognized by others. There is
limited social support or opportunity for this type of grieving, which
Leila experienced and which the letter exchange helped her to express.

As the letters evolved, Leila's relationship with the leprechaun shifted.
She began to give advice to the leprechaun on how he could deal with big
humans, who rarely recognize how terrifying their bigness can be for
little people, and to remember his many strengths despite the realities
of his current situation. Eventually a session occurred when she no longer desired communication with the leprechaun. It is my belief that Leila
moved forward in treatment having successfully expressed a range of feelings, and having had the experience of giving something (be it advice,
comfort, camaraderie, or all three) to the leprechaun. Although her future
health was uncertain, she maintained her certainty of accomplishing all of
her hopes and dreams, and later in treatment she decided that she would
become a pediatric neurologist to help children like herself.

The next stage of treatment focused on Leila's developing coping
skills to deal with the "unknowns" within her body. In an effort to
understand how Leila somatically experienced her feelings, and to show
the partnership between mind and body, we utilized the Gingerbread
Person Feelings Map (Drewes, 2001). This technique invited Leila to
identify and label her feelings, to show her affective states, and to examine the new and physically confusing feelings within her body. This
intervention was particularly effective for Leila, as she was fascinated
by anatomy. Described by her mother as "the mad scientist," Leila was
curious to learn about how and why things worked, and was eager to
find the meanings and mechanisms behind everything. Leila chose bold
colors and funky patterns, and this technique produced rich material.

Eventually writing and drawing, along with handling utensils,
became challenges for Leila as a result of her progressive impairment
in fine motor skills. In the face of these losses, both tangible (the loss

of skills) and intangible (the loss of dignity and independence), Leila's mother developed a creative strategy. One morning, noticing that the previous day Leila had been unable to hold her spoon while eating cereal, her mother decided to switch things around: She put Leila's cereal in her juice cup, poured milk (which she colored purple by combining chocolate and strawberry syrups) in her cereal bowl, and gave her a fork instead of a spoon. How silly, confusing, and incredibly ingenious this was! This strategy gave Leila the opportunity to confront her losses and to shine a light on the comedy of daily routine.

In treatment, we gently shifted our gears toward other techniques, using stuffed animals and various props rather than objects that required dexterity. In my office lived two stuffed animals with angel wings; their names were Angie and Isabeara. Leila gravitated toward Angie at the end of each session, and we decided it might be a good idea to allow Angie to take "field trips" out of the office to support Leila during her medical visits. We spent some time deciding what Angie would be permitted to do during the medical visits. This discussion allowed us to explore the rationale for certain expectations of patients (in both child and "angel" categories) during medical visits, and it enabled Leila to develop insights into her own behavior that would redefine how she presented herself during medical visits. I asked Leila how she envisioned Angie helping her, and she decided that Angie would be responsible for containing intense feelings during medical visits; on days when Leila felt capable of doing that herself, Angie would switch her role to watching for signs of "magic." The following session, Leila confidently entered the room, sat down, and asked to use the toy medical kit. I gathered the kit along with some rubber bands and gauze, and watched intently as Leila began repairing the body of Angie, whose arm had fallen off after a heated protest between Leila and the medical staff. She explained that there are just some feelings that cannot be contained, and that Angie felt a lot better after having expressed Leila's anger to the medical staff. Angie's presence resulted in a far less disruptive medical visit, and her physical injury became a tangible representation of how out of control and painful the experience of expressing strong feelings can really be. Leila empathized with the hurt Angie experienced. I told Leila that Angie's primary goal and greatest honor was to take away the pain of children. Leila stared at me for a long while and then began tenderly repairing Angie's wounds. While observing Leila's gentleness in placing Band-Aids and ointment on her fluffy patient, I also was struck by the care she took in describing complex medical terminology to the "fearful" Angie. An internal repair process was unfolding as she engaged in this powerful external repair process (Goodyear-Brown, 2010).

Our final stage of treatment highlighted Leila's resilience in the face of grief. In this stage of treatment, Leila endeavored to reclaim the magic that is characteristic of childhood. Following directives in the *Trauma-Focused Integrated Play Therapy* manual (Gil, 2011), I asked Leila to build a world in the sand tray, using as many or as few miniatures as she preferred. I explained that there was no right or wrong way to do this. She flashed a sly smile and got to work. Over the course of the next three sessions, Leila created a powerful scene within the sand tray, which she entitled the "Circle of Security." During the second session, I invited Leila to share parts of this scene by conveying a genuine curiosity about what she had created, rather than trying to interpret or problem-solve her creation. When she told me it was not yet ready, this served as a reminder that I needed to "freaking slow down." It was important to allow Leila to be the leader in defining her world in her own time.

Leila invited her mother into the room with us after the third session. Leila shared with us her world, through symbolic play, introducing us to the miniatures within the circle and the energies that we could not see. She told us that these miniatures represented ill children needing extra love, support, and protection from those around them. And when that physical demonstration of support was not enough to help these children to feel better, she decided to use "magic" sand, which she kept in special reserve for sprinkling around those in need. Her genuine desire to care for and protect others while she was struggling with her own illness is yet another beautiful and powerful example of her resilient spirit.

Signs of Resilience and Strength during the Course of Therapy

Resilience in children is not the outcome of gaining extraordinary coping skills through extraordinary means, but of developing such skills through the "everyday magic" of the children themselves, their families and friends, and their communities (Masten, 2001, 2014). Leila indeed possessed this magic. Bonanno (2004) observes that shared positive emotion and laughter are strong opponents of adversity. The spunky sense of humor that Leila and her mother shared, and their infectious laughter (which could sometimes be heard all the way down the hall from our session room), were observed to be their primary means of coping. Crenshaw (2006) once wrote, "I have always marveled at children who have experienced so much suffering and deprivation in their lives who can still manage a good sense of humor. What a treasure, what a valuable resource to sustain you through life it is, when you can see the comical and absurd side of life and have a good belly laugh once in a while" (p. 190).

Leila's personal hardiness was evident throughout her treatment as well. Writing about the grief response to intangible losses, Crenshaw and Mordock (2005), citing earlier work by Kobasa, Maddi, and Kahn (1982), explain that "hardiness" can be considered a commitment to finding a meaningful purpose to life, and to the belief that one can influence one's surroundings and grow through both positive and negative life experiences. Leila cared for and influenced the leprechaun, Angie, and the children within her "Circle of Security." As Leila regressed medically in many ways, it should be evident that she also progressed with great hardiness.

Leila's parents were important teammates in the therapeutic process. Their dedication to treatment and the genuine delight they took in their daughter on her good and bad days alike were sources of strength not only for Leila, but for me while treating Leila. They too were grieving and adjusting to many daily challenges. And yet they were consistently creative, loving, and patient with their daughter; it made perfect sense to me that this child with special needs would be cared for by parents with special qualities. Through their unconditional love and balanced perspective, Leila's parents provided a secure base for self-exploration and self-acceptance (Barnett, Clements, Kaplan-Estrin, & Fialka, 2003). The success in Leila's treatment was made possible by the involvement of these special teammates.

Leila's Inspiration through a Heartfelt Journey of Joy and Tragedy

After accepting a position at another agency in June 2013, I immediately prepared to share this news with my clients. Termination is never easy for a therapist or client, but I was especially sad about terminating treatment with Leila. By that point, though, she was coping well and engaging in treatment solely for "checkups" on a monthly basis. In truth, Leila was probably ready to terminate treatment altogether. I, on the other hand, was not. I knew that I had a lot more to learn from this child. It was 2 days before her next scheduled session when I received a phone call from her mother informing me that Leila had died in a tragic accident. I was not ready to terminate treatment, and I was certainly not ready to say goodbye.

Leila bravely accomplished her treatment goals, coping with many tangible and intangible losses in her life. Her play was rich with symbols of angels and themes of luck and hope. Throughout supervision with my Registered Play Therapy Supervisor, I was made aware of the importance of these symbols and themes and how they applied to Leila's healing process. However, it was not until I sat alone in our shared therapeutic space and reflected collectively on all of our sessions over the past 2 years that I could truly feel their power. My small office space overflowed with her radiance.

Despite the profound sense of loss that a therapist may feel when a client dies, there is minimal research on, or even conversation about, this grief. The therapist may experience elements of disenfranchised grief (Crenshaw, 2001b). This is because the therapist–client relationship is seemingly outside the scope of "permissible" grief, whereas grief in other relationships is sanctioned. As a result, the therapist may be left out of the rituals and ceremonies that are integral to celebrating the client's life and finding and giving support among a community of the client's loved ones.

Therapists build and break boundaries in an ongoing attempt to connect with clients. We invest our emotions, our time, and (quite rightly) our best selves. Leila's parents involved me in her funeral services, which permitted me to celebrate the gifts she gave me during our time together, and also permitted me to grieve alongside Leila's loved ones. This gesture had a profound impact on me, as it honored our relationship as important, emotionally rich, and real. Our relationship was seen.

Leila, in life and in death, has taught me valuable lessons. She gave gifts to a great many. In fact, months before her death she took her parents by surprise, frankly telling them to donate her organs if anything should ever happen to her. She specified that the only organs off limits were her eyes, telling her parents, "Those are mine." In the days following her death, Leila's organs saved the lives of five people.

While I believe that there can never be closure for the loss of a life as radiant as Leila's, there is always an opportunity for meaning making through shared memories and connectedness. With the collective wisdom of my family, friends, and colleagues, I have come to understand the mystery in living and in dying as both tremendously confusing and greatly comforting. As therapists, we are professionals who do the work of caring deeply, listening intently, and attaching strongly. And, when given such special opportunities, we can welcome these bright lights into our lives long after they leave the physical realm of our shared therapeutic space.

CONCLUDING COMMENTS

The resilience evident in the lives of Nick, Kara, and Leila is inspiring. Their stories are beautiful examples of Ann Masten's (2001) "ordinary magic." Expressing their grief through symbolic representation in their play and through their heartfelt poems and letters, these children actively transformed powerful feelings to create healing. When therapy works well, as it did with Leila, it is not just the client who changes, but the therapist as well. In the end, therapy is a unique and deeply human encounter; at its best, it allows for the meeting in a place and time of unbridled acceptance of the vulnerability that each human harbors but rarely risks sharing. This moment of meeting has the power to profoundly change both, so that neither will ever be the same. Could such therapy be an example of "extraordinary magic"?

REFERENCES

Axline, V. (1981). *Play therapy* (rev. ed.). New York: Ballantine Books. (Original work published 1969)

Axline, V. (1986). *Dibs in search of self*. New York: Ballantine Books. (Original work published 1964)

Balk, D. E. (1996). Models for understanding adolescents coping with bereavement. *Death Studies, 20,* 367–387.

Barnett, D., Clements, M., Kaplan-Estrin, M., & Fialka, J. (2003). Building new dreams: Supporting parents' adaptation to their child with special needs. *Infants and Young Children, 16*(3), 184–200.

Bonanno, G. A. (2004). Loss, trauma, and human resilience: Have we underestimated the human capacity to thrive after extremely aversive events? *American Psychologist, 59*(1), 20–28.

Bonanno, G. A. (2009). *The other side of sadness: What the new science of bereavement tells us about life after loss*. New York: Basic Books.

Bonanno, G. A., & Diminich, E. D. (2013). Annual research review: Positive adjustment to adversity—Trajectories of minimal-impact resilience and emergent resilience. *Journal of Child Psychology Psychiatry, 54*(4), 378–401.

Blanco, P. J., Muro, J. H., & Stickley, V. K. (2014). Understanding the concept of genuineness in play therapy: Implications for the supervision and teaching of beginning play therapists. *International Journal of Play Therapy, 23*(1), 44–54.

Brooks, R. B., & Goldstein, S. (2001). *Raising resilient children: Fostering strength, hope and optimism in our children*. New York: McGraw-Hill.

Brooks, R. B., & Goldstein, S. (2003). *Nurturing resilience in our children: Answers to the most important parenting questions*. New York: McGraw-Hill.

Brown, S. (2009). *Play: How it shapes the brain, opens the imagination, and invigorates the soul*. New York: Avery/Penguin.

Cohen, J. A., & Mannarino, A. P. (2010). Trauma-focused cognitive behavioral therapy for traumatized children and adolescents. *European Psychotherapy, 9*(1), 69–80.

Crenshaw, D. A. (1990). *Bereavement: Counseling the grieving throughout the life cycle.* New York: Continuum.

Crenshaw, D. A. (2001a). The disenfranchised grief of children. In K. J. Doka (Ed.), *Disenfranchised grief: New directions, challenges and strategies for practice* (pp. 293–306). Champaign, IL: Research Press.

Crenshaw, D. A. (2001b). Party hats on monsters. In H. G. Kaduson & C. E. Schaefer (Eds.), *101 more favorite play therapy techniques* (pp. 124–127). Northvale, NJ: Jason Aronson.

Crenshaw, D. A. (2006). *Evocative strategies in child and adolescent psychotherapy.* Lanham, MD: Jason Aronson.

Crenshaw, D. A. (2013). A resilience framework for treating severe childhood trauma. In S. Goldstein & R. B. Brooks (Eds.), *Handbook of resilience in children* (2nd ed., pp. 309–328). New York: Springer.

Crenshaw, D. A., & Kenney-Noziska, S. (2014). Therapeutic presence in play therapy. *International Journal of Play Therapy, 23*(1), 31–43.

Crenshaw, D. A., & Mordock, J. B. (2005). *Understanding and treating the aggression of children: Fawns in gorilla suits.* Lanham, MD: Jason Aronson.

Drewes, A. A. (2001). The Gingerbread Person Feelings Map. In H. G. Kaduson & C. E. Schaefer (Eds.), *101 more favorite play therapy techniques* (pp. 92–97). Northvale, NJ: Jason Aronson.

Drewes, A. A. (2011a). Integrating play therapy theories into practice. In A. A. Drewes, S. C. Bratton, & C. E. Schaefer (Eds.), *Integrative play therapy* (pp. 21–35). Hoboken, NJ: Wiley.

Drewes, A. A. (2011b). Integrative play therapy. In C. E. Schaeffer (Ed.), *Foundations of play therapy* (2nd ed., pp. 349–364). Hoboken, NJ: Wiley.

Drewes, A. A., Bratton, S. C., & Schaefer, C. E. (Eds.). (2011). *Integrative play therapy.* Hoboken, NJ: Wiley.

Fredrickson, B. (2004). The broaden-and-build theory of positive emotion. *Philosophical Transactions of the Royal Society of London: Series B. Biological Sciences, 359,* 1367–1377.

Fuller, A., McGraw, K., & Goodyear, M. (2002). Bungy jumping through life: A developmental framework for the promotion of resilience. In L. Rowling, G. Martin, & L. Walker (Eds.), *Mental health promotion and young people: Concepts and practice* (pp. 84–96). Sydney: McGraw-Hill Australia.

Gaskill, R. L., & Perry, B. D. (2014). The neurobiological power of play: Using the Neurosequential Model of Therapeutics to guide play in the healing process. In C. A. Malchiodi & D. A. Crenshaw (Eds.), *Creative arts and play therapy for attachment problems* (pp. 178–194). New York: Guilford Press.

Gil, E. (1991). *Healing power of play: Working with abused children.* New York: Guilford Press.

Gil, E. (2006). *Helping abused and traumatized children: Integrating directive and nondirective approaches.* New York: Guilford Press.

Gil, E. (2010). *Working with children to heal interpersonal trauma: The power of play.* New York: Guilford Press.

Gil, E. (2011). *Trauma-focused integrated play therapy (TF IPT): An evidence- and practice-informed treatment model for working with traumatized children.* Manual presented at the Play Therapy Works Summer Seminar, Eastham, MA.

Gil, E. (2014). The creative use of metaphor in play and art therapy with attachment problems. In C. A. Malchiodi & D. A. Crenshaw (Eds.), *Creative arts and play therapy for attachment problems* (pp. 159–177). New York: Guilford Press

Goodyear-Brown, P. (2010). *Play therapy with traumatized children: A prescriptive approach.* Hoboken, NJ: Wiley.

Goldstein, S., & Brooks, R. B. (2013). Why study resilience? In S. Goldstein & R. B. Brooks (Eds.), *Handbook of resilience in children* (2nd ed., pp. 3–14). New York: Springer.

James, B. (1989). *Treating traumatized children.* Boston: Lexington Books.

James, B. (1994). *Handbook for treatment of attachment-trauma problems in children.* New York: Lexington Books.

Kobasa, S. C., Maddi, S. R., & Kahn, S. (1982). Hardiness and health: A prospective study. *Journal of Personality and Social Psychology, 42,* 168–172.

Landreth, G. L. (1982). *Play therapy: Dynamics of counseling with children.* Springfield, IL: Charles C Thomas.

Landreth, G. L. (2002). *Play therapy: The art of the relationship* (2nd ed.). New York: Brunner-Routledge.

Landreth, G. L. (2012). *Play therapy: The art of the relationship* (3rd ed.). New York: Brunner-Routledge.

Lin, K., Sandler, I., Ayers, T., Wolchik, S., & Laucken, L. (2004). Resilience in parentally bereaved children and adolescents seeking preventative services. *Journal of Clinical Child and Adolescent Psychology, 33,* 673–683.

Mannarino, A. P., & Cohen, J. A. (2011). Traumatic loss in children and adolescents. *Journal of Child and Adolescent Trauma, 4*(1), 22–33.

Masten, A. S. (2001). Ordinary magic: Resilience processes in development. *American Psychologist, 56*(3), 227–238.

Masten, A. S. (2014). *Ordinary magic: Resilience in development.* New York: Guilford Press.

Masten, A. S., & Narayan, A.J. (2012). Child development in the context of disaster, war, and terrorism: Pathways of risk and resilience. *Annual Review of Psychology, 63,* 227–257.

Mills, J. C., & Crowley, R. J. (1986). *Therapeutic metaphors for children and the child within.* New York: Brunner-Routledge.

Mills, J. C., & Crowley, R. J. (2014). *Therapeutic metaphors for children and the child within* (2nd ed.). New York: Brunner-Routledge.

Moustakas, C. (1953). *Children in play therapy.* New York: McGraw-Hill.

Moustakas, C. (1959). *Psychotherapy with children.* New York: Harper.

Moustakas, C. (1997). *Relationship play therapy.* Northvale, NJ: Jason Aronson.

Rogers, C. R. (1957). The necessary and sufficient conditions of therapeutic personality change. *Journal of Consulting Psychology, 21,* 97–103.

Rogers, C. R. (1980). *A way of being.* Boston: Houghton Mifflin.

Rogers, C. R., & Truax, C. B. (1976). The therapeutic conditions antecedent to change: A theoretical view. In C. R. Rogers, E. T. Gendlin, D. J. Kiesler, & C. B. Truax (Eds.), *The therapeutic relationship and its impact: A study of psychotherapy with schizophrenics* (pp. 97–108). Westport, CT: Greenwood Press.

Rutter, M. (2006). Implications of resilience concepts for scientific understanding. *Annals of the New York Academy of Sciences, 1094,* 1–12.

Schaefer, C. E. (Ed.). (1993). *The therapeutic powers of play.* Northvale, NJ: Jason Aronson.

Schaefer, C. E., & Drewes, A. A. (Eds.). (2013). *The therapeutic powers of play: 20 core agents of change* (2nd ed.). Hoboken, NJ: Wiley.

Schore, A. N. (2012). *The science and art of psychotherapy.* New York: Norton.

Seymour, J. W. (2014). Integrated play therapy with childhood traumatic grief. In C. A. Malchiodi & D. A. Crenshaw (Eds.), *Creative arts and play therapy for attachment problems* (pp. 259–274). New York: Guilford Press.

Shelby, J. S. (2010). Cognitive-behavioral therapy and play therapy for childhood trauma and loss. In N. B. Webb (Ed.), *Helping bereaved children: A handbook for practitioners* (3rd ed., pp. 263–277). New York: Guilford Press.

Shelby, J. S., & Felix, E. D. (2005). Posttraumatic play therapy: The need for an integrated model of directive and nondirective approaches. In L. A. Reddy, T. M. Files-Hall, & C. E. Schaefer (Eds.), *Empirically based play interventions for children* (pp. 79–103). Washington, DC: American Psychological Association.

Siegel, D. J. (2012). *The developing mind: How relationships and the brain interact to shape who we are.* New York: Guilford Press.

Steele, W., & Machiodi, C. A. (Eds.). (2012). *Trauma-informed practices with children and adolescents.* New York: Routledge.

Stokes, J. A. (2007). Resilience and bereaved children: Helping a child to develop a resilient mind-set following the death of Donne parent. In B. Munroe & D. Oliviere (Eds.), *Resilience in palliative care: Achieving in adversity* (pp. 39–65). Oxford, UK: Oxford University Press.

Terr, E. (1991). Childhood traumas. *American Journal of Psychiatry, 148,* 10–20.

van der Kolk, B. A., Spinazzola, J., Blaustein, M. E., Hopper, J. W., Hopper, E. K., Korn, D. L., et al. (2007). A randomized clinical trial of eye movement desensitization and reprocessing (EMDR), fluoxetine, and pill placebo in the treatment of posttraumatic stress disorder: Treatment effects and long-term maintenance. *Journal of Clinical Psychiatry, 68*(1), 37–46.

Webb, N. B. (Ed.). (2007). *Play therapy with children in crisis: A casebook for practitioners* (3rd ed). New York: Guilford Press.

Webb, N. B. (Ed.). (2010). *Helping bereaved children: A handbook for practitioners* (3rd ed.). New York: Guilford Press.

Wolin, S., & Wolin, S. J. (1996). The challenge model: Working with the strengths of children of substance abusing parents. *Child and Adolescent Psychiatric Clinics of North America, 5*(1), 243–256.

Wolin, S. J., & Wolin, S. (1992). The challenge model: How children rise above adversity. *Family Dynamics of Addiction Quarterly, 2*(2), 10–22.

Wolin, S. J., & Wolin, S. (1993). *The resilient self: How survivors of troubled families rise above adversity.* New York: Villard Books.

Chapter 5

Posttraumatic Play

A Robust Path to Resilience

ELIANA GIL

THE NATURE OF POSTTRAUMATIC PLAY

Posttraumatic play has been well documented as a unique form of play that children initiate after traumatic events—sometimes on their own, and other times after being encouraged to do so in a clinical setting (Dripchak, 2007; Gil, 2010; Marvasti, 1994; Schaefer, 1994; Terr, 1991). It has a noble intent: to help children regain mastery over traumatic experiences. It is also a very pure, original, and intuitive form of self-help; children often arrive at this type of play organically. In fact, Dripchak (2007) notes that the child "both guides and is guided by the play therapy process" (p. 127).

Our current knowledge base about the impact of trauma, and about ways of assisting those who endure trauma, has grown vastly in the last two decades—so much so that a degree of consensus now exists about where clinical effort should be directed, although there is still ample discussion of how to achieve those goals. At its most basic level, treatment of trauma seeks to facilitate the following:

1. Identification and acknowledgment of the traumatic stressor.
2. Expression of thoughts, feelings, and sensations about the impact of the stressor.
3. Opportunities to regain mastery and control.
4. Discharge, release, or mobility (to combat the usual freeze–flight–fight responses).

5. Development of a cohesive narrative with a beginning, middle, and end.
6. Movement forward (disengagement from traumatic material).

Children's posttraumatic play achieves these aims in a distinctive fashion, most familiar to, and valued by, those trained in play therapy and other expressive arts. Play therapists recognize the inherent curative factors in play—those that allow children to externalize what is on their minds—in an effort to gain a safe enough distance from which to begin addressing and managing their concerns. Posttraumatic play has several characteristics, including its tendency to be literal play; to be repetitive; to be joyless and noninteractive, especially at first; and quite often, a tendency to look rigid in its repetition, with microscopic changes signaling that curative factors of management are beginning to emerge (Terr, 1981). (When such changes do not occur, this is an indication that the play may be toxic rather than dynamic in nature; I discuss this distinction further below, as well as how to assist a child who seems "stuck" in toxic play.)

There are two fundamental aspects of posttraumatic play. First, it is instinctive in children, and they often initiate and manage the play on their own (as noted above). Even when they don't, clinicians are often surprised and delighted by how receptive children are to engaging in posttraumatic play when provided with literal symbols of the traumatic experiences. Posttraumatic play is children's invention, congruent with their desire to express themselves, make meaning, and strive toward mastery. Second, posttraumatic play ideally occurs in the presence of an unconditional witness—someone who "holds" the child's experience without judgment, does not look away, and gently welcomes whatever the child needs to bring forward. Children who utilize posttraumatic play effectively are demonstrating trust in the therapist/witness and a wish for all their thoughts and feelings to be accepted by others. This may be a biologically driven need for emotional connection. During a keynote speech that I attended, Daniel Siegel made the statement, "Brains are hard-wired to look for other brains, to find connections." The unconditional witness also provides the companionship that often eludes traumatized children, who are often embedded in others' secrecy, in danger, or in a lack of available resources.

All these inherent trials make it all the more remarkable that children often push ahead to start posttraumatic play, which I strongly believe not only enhances but is powered by children's resilience. The following case illustration vividly demonstrates how children can survive and thrive after overwhelming traumatic stressors.

CLINICAL CASE EXAMPLE:
ALLYSON AND STEPHANIE

When I think about this child and her mother, I remember the intense vicarious traumatization I experienced; their situation caused me no end of consternation and despair. However, my next immediate memory is the feeling of awe that welled up in me as I served as an unconditional witness to a resilient child's way of acknowledging, externalizing, exploring, expressing, and managing her overwhelming experiences. This case asserted what I hold dear and true in my heart: Children have remarkable capacities to recognize and access inner resources and to use those resources on their own behalf. In this case, the child's posttraumatic play was an unmistakable marker of her resilience and yielded great benefits. This case also demonstrates the need for retaining a contextual framework in working with traumatized children, as well as making a clinical investment in anchoring therapy in a consistent, predictable, and empathic therapeutic relationship with children and their caregivers.

Referral and First Meeting

Four-year-old Allyson and her mother, Stephanie, were referred by an astute preschool teacher who had heard that the mother had undergone an intensely traumatic event and the child had witnessed it. The child's behavior had regressed in the preschool setting after this event, and the teacher described Allyson as "unsettled, emotional, and often inconsolable." When Allyson came into therapy, she was energetic, easily distracted, and unable to focus on any one thing for very long. However, she separated easily from her mother, a petite 26-year-old Hispanic woman who looked frail and pale.

Stephanie brought her young daughter to our first meeting, even though I had made it clear to her that the intake session was best done without the child present, so that the mother (or other caregiver) could feel comfortable speaking freely. Stephanie said she was not able to come alone, reportedly because her daughter was not tolerating separations from her mother at this time. Allyson's independent behavior made me question her mother's explanation about why she had brought her daughter to the intake appointment. This explanation that did not ring true was the first hint that Stephanie was keeping Allyson nearby to comfort her, not the other way around.

Allyson ran into the play therapy room, and I suggested to Stephanie that I meet with her daughter and that she return when Allyson was in preschool, so that we could speak alone. She complied with this request.

Intake Meeting with the Mother

A week later, when Stephanie came back to talk with me, she cried from the moment she sat down until she left. This caused me to decide to schedule some time to see the mother as well as her daughter (at different times of the week, but in parallel fashion). Stephanie seemed relieved to be able to speak in Spanish. She seemed to find it easy to talk to me in earnest, stating that she could only do so because she could speak in her mother tongue. She told me that she had been to a non-Spanish-speaking therapist prior to seeing me, but she found the stress of going through a translator more than she could bear. Thus I agreed to see her; I felt that I could work with both separately, but hoped to bring them together at some point. Stephanie was unemployed and thus able to attend weekly sessions for both her daughter and herself.

Stephanie seemed very concerned about Allyson, but detached at the same time. She expressed feeling worried about her, but could not organize her thoughts enough to express her specific concerns. Over the next 2 months, Stephanie and Allyson began to show and tell components of their traumatic experience, since neither was able to give an organized narrative with congruent emotional responses. At times when the mother talked about the trauma, she spoke in a flat tone, as if she was describing something that had happened to someone in a story. At other times, her emotionality seemed overwhelming and she sobbed uncontrollably; she was clearly experiencing the hyperarousal and numbing consistent with posttraumatic stress disorder, and yet was unable to articulate words and sentences about what she had endured.

Stephanie was able to communicate that she had been raped for 12 hours while Allyson was both awake and asleep in the next room. She told me that Allyson had peeked in from the door and run back to her room. Stephanie noted that when the ordeal began, she wanted to protect her daughter from getting hurt by the rapist; however, by the time it was over, she simply did not have the energy to care what happened to her daughter (she said this dispassionately). Stephanie had sent Allyson to the next-door neighbor after the rapist left their apartment, and the distressed neighbor had called the police and ambulance. Stephanie was taken to the emergency room, while Allyson was put in the custody of the police and later in emergency foster placement.

When we discussed the police and mental health services in more detail, Stephanie said that she had talked to someone the police had brought to her house. She said it was not helpful to talk to someone who also cried with her about what had happened. Stephanie told me she had seen this counselor about six times with a translator, but didn't remember most of it and felt that "the lady was not strong enough to listen" to her. Stephanie told me that Allyson had also talked to a counselor after the rape, but she had "mostly played" and seemed happy, which gave Stephanie the impression that she had probably not "understood what she saw," had not "seen anything bad," or "forgot it already." The mother's denial was expectable: She didn't deny that the child had looked into the room while she was being raped, but she denied the impact of that experience, hoping to help herself by reassuring herself that her child was happy and had likely forgotten the traumatic event already.

The specific details of Stephanie's sexual assault are not described here, in order to prevent readers from feeling vicarious traumatization. Suffice to say that the details of this Type 1 trauma (an acute event) were horrifying, and it was necessary for Stephanie to organize her thoughts and feelings about the traumatic event in order to feel that she had faced it sufficiently to regain personal control. "I don't want this to define who I am from here on out," she shared with me once, adding, "I don't want it messing with my head when I'm doing something else, I want to think about it only when I want to think about it." These statements reflected Stephanie's personal drive toward health. It is worth noting, however, that this Type 1 trauma was further exacerbated by Stephanie's family and social context, in which support systems were few and far between. The extended family seemed remarkably nonempathic—in fact, judgmental that Stephanie had chosen to live in an unsafe neighborhood and had opened her door to a stranger. Her extended family thus added unwanted pressure, increased Stephanie's already substantial sense of guilt, and interfered with her recovery. Stephanie's mother went as far as to suggest that she had tempted the man into rape by opening the door and inviting him in when he asked to use her phone. She insisted that Stephanie go to church and confess her sins; this made Stephanie feel as if she could not go to her church or take part in its social activities because she could not bring herself to confess her sins.

Therapeutic Approaches to Posttraumatic Play

Stephanie's trauma work took the form of direct gradual exposure, which has been described as a treatment of choice for rape survivors (Foa & Rothbaum, 1998). This cognitive-behavioral approach to processing rape is comforting in its structure and direction, and, as strenuous as it is, it produces positive results in a definitive manner for adults. However, this approach is not proven to work with children, whose cognitive and linguistic limitations compromise its usefulness.

Children appear to have unique opportunities for processing traumatic events—in fact, more ample opportunities than adults have, since children are not limited to verbal processing. Although spontaneous verbalization of traumatic memories can often accompany the play of traumatized children, it is not required or demanded. In fact, clinicians who are trained in play therapy (especially child-centered play therapy), value play therapy for its many inherent curative properties, not simply as a way to get children comfortable or prepare them to talk (Ray, 2011). I value and lead with child-centered play therapy in many cases of child therapy addressing childhood trauma; however, some traumatized children can be quite hesitant to process traumatic material at first and may need clinical direction or encouragement to do so. Thus, for decades, I have used an integrative approach that incorporates nondirective and directive approaches. With this approach, I have learned firsthand what children can accomplish in their play, with or without clinical prodding (Gil, 2007, 2010). Specifically, furnishing toys that provide literal representation of aspects of the trauma can serve as gentle encouragement to traumatized children. Having said that, I concur with Shelby and Felix (2005), who state: "In cases in which a child replays the traumatic event without prompting, the self-initiated posttraumatic play may be advantageous over therapist-directed posttraumatic play by providing the perception of increased control over content, pacing, and mode of expression and exploration" (p. 84).

Given the specific details of this case and what Allyson witnessed, it is relevant to note that research on play therapy with children who have witnessed domestic violence has shown an increase in positive self-concept and a decrease in externalizing behaviors (Kot, 1996; Kot & Tyndall-Lind, 2005; Tyndall-Lind, 1999). These positive outcomes make a major contribution to a sense of mastery and restoration of control. DeMaria and Cowden (1992) also encourage the use of play therapy, stating that "changes in self-concept must be achieved indirectly, through the child's experiences, activities, and environment, thus allowing the child to experience him- or herself in a new way. In turn, the child has the chance to create new beliefs about her potential and abilities" (p. 41).

Dynamic versus Toxic Posttraumatic Play

As I have noted earlier in this chapter, I consider posttraumatic play one of the best indicators that resilience exists in a child to begin with. The intent of posttraumatic play is to give traumatized children opportunities to face and conquer their fears in order to achieve mastery. One could say that resilience is the "wind beneath the wings" of posttraumatic play. However, not all children embrace and/or spontaneously implement such play, and Terr (1981), the first person to chronicle this type of play, cautions that it can sometimes become dangerous if its original intent of mastery is not achieved.

Elsewhere, I have discussed the difference between "dynamic" and "toxic" posttraumatic play; the latter presents unique concerns and challenges (Gil, 2010). Even so, the fact that children are initiating this type of play is promising, and the toxic play can be moved forward (once it is identified and addressed) in a more directive way. I have thought about this for years, and my perception is that the play becomes "stuck" or toxic when the repetitive play remains rigid, stays strictly sequential, and brings about no differences in affective status or outcome. What appears to cause this lack of mobility is that the posttraumatic play, which usually provides a safe enough distance, fails to provide that cushion of safety. Instead, it's possible that these children feel so connected and close to the posttraumatic play that they can feel retraumatized. This occurs because their play causes "revivification"— a reliving (rather than remembering) of the event. Revivification is a process by which an event is brought back to life, and in this case overpowers a child's intent of mastery, by placing the child back in the original situation physiologically, emotionally, and psychologically.

One of my young clients had experienced surgery in the context of neglectful parents who had left her alone to fend for herself. She initiated posttraumatic play as a means to address her debilitating helplessness when she found herself alone and ill (and, later, acutely afraid) in a hospital. However, her play became revivifying and was insufficient to buffer her; instead, her sensation was that she was having surgery over and over again. In fact, her foster parents reported that she would complain of acute pain in her surgical scar, similar to the pain she endured when she was placed in postoperative care. For this little client, it became imperative that she remember and address her intense fears regarding the surgery (and parental abandonment) in such a way that she could eventually achieve the necessary distance to process her trauma and reach a position of mastery and control.

I have struggled to find useful interventions in cases of revivifying play. The most successful ones have involved creating an additional cushion of safety by placing the play one dimension farther away (out of touch). For example, the clinician can video-record the posttraumatic play and show it back to the child on the screen. Another idea is to use an actual mirror, placing it near the posttraumatic play (dollhouse, sand tray, drawing) so that the child sees the image of the play. Children who are unfortunately stuck in their posttraumatic play may find themselves able to restore the reparative aspects of the posttraumatic play in these ways. These and other ways of intervening are discussed in Gil (2010).

Among the most consistent questions about posttraumatic play are how long it should be allowed to continue uninterrupted and how to know whether it is dynamic or toxic play. Answering these questions requires clinical attention to detail and the use of active observation. In fact, small details should be chronicled so that subtle changes (in sequence, characters, storylines, placement of the play, etc.) can signal that the play is dynamic. Conversely, toxic posttraumatic play persists as repetitive, noninteractional play, with literally no changes in process or content. It is important for clinicians to consistently assess posttraumatic play's progress toward the intended goals of mastery and restoration of control.

Allyson's Individual Therapy

Allyson was slow to warm up to posttraumatic play. From the moment she came into our first unscheduled meeting, she was quite dysregulated— jumping, making guttural sounds, throwing things, moving all around the room, coming up to me and making faces, spitting, and so on. My initial work with her was being patient, accepting, anchored, and open to all her interactions—that is, providing the permissive environment of child-centered play therapy (Axline, 1969; Landreth, 1991). At the same time, as a practitioner of trauma-informed, integrated play therapy who was acutely aware of this child's anxiety and suffering, I also immediately began to consider some strategies designed to help her regulate her emotions. One day when she was jumping up and down, I placed a Biodot* on her skin and focused her on what color it would become when placed on her hand. (I waited until she was quite agitated, so that the Biodot would reflect the intense emotion immediately.) She then became intrigued when I told her I could show her a way to change the color. She was receptive to a breathing exercise and listening to soft music for about 3 minutes. When we looked at her Biodot, it had changed colors, and she found this exciting. Her ability to focus long enough to change the color was short-lived, however.

---

* Biodots are small, round dots that function in the same way as "mood rings": They turn different colors, depending on the temperature of the skin. They are available at *www.biodots.org* and serve as an inexpensive way to help children with affect regulation.

Another time I had some bubbles in the room, and I asked her to watch me blow little bubbles as well as large ones, depending on how big the breath was that I took. I asked her to try it herself, but she was unable to focus enough to take deep breaths and blow out slowly or quickly. I changed the bubble activity so that I would blow the bubbles and she would clap her hands and pop them. This Theraplay activity (Booth & Jernberg, 2010) proceeds into a fun activity in which children use their knees, elbows, foreheads, toes, or other body parts to pop the bubbles. This was an activity that Allyson liked to do often, and it tired her out. After this aerobic activity, we made a game out of being very tired and needing to have some "fresh lemonade" in a little cup. During these early sessions, she also picked up and examined a lot of toys and games, but could not direct her attention to any one thing long enough to stick with an activity to its conclusion.

In our sixth session, Allyson moved over to the sand box and began to put some objects in the center of the tray. She put in two fenced-in areas, one larger than the other. Inside one of the fences, she placed a sleeping baby; in the other, she placed a dog with three heads (a figure from the Harry Potter series), as well as a woman in a bathing suit who was leaning back on her elbows. At first, Allyson simply placed the woman in the tray. Later on, she began to place her head down with her buttocks exposed. She spent quite a bit of time with these two fenced-in areas and moved the objects around in the tray. I reflected that there were two fenced-in areas, separate from each other—one with a baby, and one with a woman and a three-headed dog. "That dog has three heads," she told me. "I see," I responded, and then she said that the dog "has eight eyes!" but after counting them, she revised this to "six eyes." She later offered that the dog was a "guard dog" and could "kill people."

The work/play that Allyson did was very slow and purposeful at this juncture, and to an untrained eye, it could have looked random and inconsequential. In fact, something very substantial was taking place: Allyson was beginning to take the first step in her healing journey. She was externalizing the traumatic event as she experienced it, and in the most articulate way she had available—through the language of play. Her mother had been trapped in one room with an unknown, threatening person. She had been trapped in another room, her own; she left and returned to this room at will, but the room made her feel trapped nevertheless, as well as helpless and alone.

During the next 2 months, Allyson played in the sand box seemingly without rhyme or reason: She approached the sand box in a discontinuous fashion, at will. I maintained a nondirective approach except when I gave her some specific directives about relaxation or guided imagery, or when she needed redirecting because her intense emotions elicited erratic physical responses that seemed to be out of her control. For example, I used the sound of a chime to get her attention and asked her to listen to the chime with her eyes shut until she could no longer hear it. During this time, I asked her to breathe in and out slowly while she listened. Because Allyson was receptive to this brief exercise, I also introduced an age-appropriate story that she would listen to with her eyes closed. The story was guided imagery about a little insect who explored the forest and eventually found "just the right safe place," in which she could read, sunbathe under a sun lamp, cook up delicious broths, and listen to her favorite music. Allyson's favorite part of this story was when the little insect, usually a ladybug, could invite in a friend she liked to share marshmallows with. She usually picked a "really nice spider" or "a very small butterfly" to come into the safe space with her little insect. This guided imagery became a resource that Allyson later shared with her mother at nighttime.

I also began to understand Allyson's relentless need to come in and out of my office, presumably checking on her mother in the waiting room. As I watched her come and go, I realized that she was having an unconscious behavioral reenactment—a behavioral attempt to advance her sense of mastery. Sometimes when she saw her mother in the waiting room, she would go and climb into her lap. The mother always seemed surprised and embarrassed by her daughter's behavior, and initially she would rise and try to lead her back into the therapy room. Eventually, however, Stephanie talked to me about her daughter's behavior in the office and said that she had given it some thought. (I always supported Stephanie's thinking about Allyson's behavior as a message of some kind. I had asked her to think of her daughter's behaviors, especially those she didn't understand initially, as ways that Allyson was expressing a need she could not verbalize. The mother took this advice seriously, often sharing her insights.) Regarding Allyson's behavior in the office, which had embarrassed her initially since she didn't see other children doing it, Stephanie shared with me: "It might be that she just wants to come out to this room and check in on me, make sure I'm not being hurt." I could not contain my excitement as I said to her, "Wow, that is a great insight you've had! You are really getting to know your daughter better and better. You're really tuned in to her." Stephanie liked hearing this, and she smiled.

Throughout Allyson's repetitive posttraumatic play, I remained committed to keeping her safe from throwing toys around the office or at me. I also began to document when her emotional dysregulation became the most intense. I was able to chronicle and define that her dysregulation accompanied her activity in the sand box and the creation of her play narrative. Over time, she was able to contain the dysregulation by getting hugs from her mother, by sitting in a stuffed pillow and cradling a large stuffed rabbit, or by winding up a toy that played soft and rhythmic music.

The sand therapy was evolving as well. The two small containers persisted in the sand trays that she made, and the female figure was exposed to one degree or another as the baby began to wander outside the little container. I said to her, "The baby comes in and out of his space." "That's *her* room," she shared, almost annoyed with me that I had guessed wrong. "I see," adding, "That's a little girl who has a room, and she's coming and going." Allyson then looked up and said in a whisper, "She's trying to help her mommy, but she can't." "Oh," I repeated, "the little girl is trying to help her mommy, but she can't." "She's too little," Allyson said. "Of course," I stated. "I can tell that the little girl is very little. She can't really help her mommy even if she wants to." "Yeah," Allyson said, "and her mommy tells her to go back to her room all the time." "Oh," I repeated, "Mommy is telling her to go to her room."

Within a few months of sporadic sand therapy, Allyson created a narrative of what had happened to her mom ("The mean man hurt her and made her cry and scream. I covered my ears"); what she (Allyson) had done ("I hid under the bed, then I cried a lot, then I kept looking to see if the bad man was gone"); and what happened next ("My mommy had blood, and the blood was on the bed and the floor, and it got on my PJs"). Allyson also told me that the police came to get them, and her mom had to go to the hospital, and she had to go stay with Bill and Kate (the emergency foster parents). At one point I wondered out loud, "I wonder how the police knew to come help." "I know!" Allyson said excitedly, "I went to Leila's house and told her my mommy was hurt. She called the police." "Wow, Allyson," I said, "so even though you were little and didn't know what to do, and felt scared, you figured out to get help for your mommy. You helped after all." "That was me," Allyson said. "I was scared and ran fast." "So you were scared and ran fast," I reflected. "Yeah," she said, completely still and available. "I was scared and made my legs move fast." "I can see that," I repeated. "You were scared and made your legs move fast. Wow. You helped your mommy by running as fast as you could." She said quickly, "Watch this," and bolted out of the room to the waiting room, announcing to Stephanie, "My legs move fast." Stephanie held her daughter in her arms and said, "Yes, they do." Stephanie did not really have a reference for this statement, but by now she was feeling more prepared to give her daughter the affirmations she needed.

Parallel Trauma-Focused Treatment of Mother and Daughter

During the course of treatment with Allyson and with Stephanie, I was mindful of the parallel track that existed in this case: Both individuals (mother and child) had to process their experiences in their own unique ways, and in whatever ways felt right to each. Stephanie was able to process her traumatic memories in a structured way, using cognitive-behavioral approaches. The work was undertaken when Stephanie had developed good coping strategies and knew how to slow down or stop the conversation when she felt overwhelmed with emotion. I had given her a copy of a handout that listed expectable responses by rape survivors (Foa & Rothbaum, 1998); she read and reread this information, gleaning a deeper understanding of what she had endured and how others typically cope. Stephanie was able to see that some of her early symptoms were improving, and this caused her to feel relieved. Following Foa and Rothbaum's (1998) expert advice, I helped Stephanie approach her rape trauma via gradual exposure strategies, encouraging her release of affect and cognitive processing. She cried as she wove together her many flashbacks, organizing her memories into a coherent timeline. She remembered forgotten details, and she found her voice, putting words to the fear and rage she felt toward the rapist. She reached her stride as she confronted the rapist (through guided imagery and role playing) for allowing her young daughter to see what was going on. In some ways, Stephanie was more indignant about the rapist's disregard of Allyson than she was about what he had done to herself. Stephanie seemed afraid or reluctant to feel or express rage toward the rapist; she later shared the insight that she "didn't want to feel emotions that could lead her to want to kill someone," which was a sin in her church. During these cognitive reviews, Stephanie also acknowledged how she helped and protected Allyson by sending her back to her room and begging the rapist to spare her daughter.

But clearly there were issues related to the rape's being witnessed by her daughter that caused additional complications in Stephanie's recovery. The guilt she felt at surrendering to sleep at the end of the rape, once the man pulled away from her and left the apartment, was intense. She felt that at that point she should have mobilized herself to keep her daughter safe and to comfort her, but she simply did not have the strength she would have needed to do this, and it was likely that she actually passed out. Luckily, this man ignored the child in her room and left quickly once he decided to take flight. By then, Allyson had heightened sensory experiences and had heard him walk out, and after she tried to wake her mom to no avail, she ran to get the neighbor.

Stephanie had never had a clear sense of how her story had evolved, how much Allyson had seen, how to talk to her daughter about what had happened, or what Allyson's needs were in this regard. In the months that had passed since the rape, Stephanie had literally told Allyson to "forget what happened" and "move on." Allyson had not had much opportunity to process what she had seen, heard, sensed, and imagined, so her dysregulated behavior seemed to have an important function, since it continued to signal her distress. The clinical invitation in the play therapy office was for Allyson to find ways of showing herself (and me) what had happened and how she felt. Multiple times, I asked Allyson about the baby girl and what she was thinking or how she felt. Sometimes Allyson responded; sometimes she did not, instead staring into space (which I interpreted as brief dissociative responses). Eventually, as she felt comfortable, what needed to come forward did, in its own unique way. Sometimes Allyson "owned" what she had seen, heard, and done, and other times she used the "safe enough distance" of the little girl she had placed in her sand tray. It was particularly interesting to note that the feeling Allyson most avoided and displaced was her anger toward her mother. I'm not even sure Allyson knew what caused her anger, but the anger was embodied and electrifying. In one session, Allyson, with the little girl in her hand, yelled at the mom figure, "Get up, get up, punch him, run . . . " and in this way implied that she felt anger at her mother for not fighting to protect them both from the trauma. (I made a clinical note to include two goals in the conjoint therapy with Stephanie and Allyson: encouraging Allyson to express her fear and anger directly to her mother; and helping Stephanie accept the anger, depersonalize it, and provide the reassurance and comfort she had not been able to provide to Allyson during the traumatic event.)

The parallel process of trauma-focused work had progressed well with Stephanie and Allyson thus far, and I had kept Stephanie informed about her daughter's progress and how well she was utilizing posttraumatic play. Stephanie, in turn, kept me abreast of how Allyson was doing at home. Some of her initial concerns had subsided, since Allyson seemed less clingy, more self-assured, and less reactive to other children.

When I first talk to parents about play therapy and what therapy will look like for their children, I invite them to do a simple expressive therapy activity, such as a play genogram, a sand tray, or a drawing. I invited Stephanie to participate in these activities. Even though she went to the sand box and moved the sand around, sifting it between her fingers, she much preferred talking to nonverbal communication, so her investment in sand therapy (or other expressive therapies) was initially very ambivalent.

The Rationale for Conjoint Sessions

I told both Allyson and Stephanie that we were going to have some time together in the same room, at the same time, so that Allyson and Stephanie could take a look at this very difficult event that they had experienced together. The hope was that by doing so, they would feel stronger (and possibly closer). At this point, my goal was to help mother and daughter co-create a narrative and share their perspectives in a way that would be age-appropriate for Allyson and would emphasize mastery. I had coached the mother about creating a safe and supportive environment with unconditional acceptance of Allyson's play and behavior. I encouraged her to look for, and emphasize, any thoughts, feelings, or behaviors that were consistent with Allyson's mastery of her traumatic experience.

I had two specific objectives in conducting these conjoint sessions. First, I wanted to give Stephanie and Allyson a chance to present their individually created narratives to each other, so that their experiences of the traumatic assault could be shared and acknowledged. Second, because both Stephanie and Allyson had experienced profound helplessness and fear, it would be important for Allyson to change her perception of Stephanie as incapable of protecting herself and Allyson in the future. In fact, one of the desired outcomes of treatment with children who have witnessed their mothers beaten or abused is restoring the parents to the role of capable and nurturing protectors (Lieberman & van Horn, 2004). Once the children are helped to reestablish their perception of the parents as shielding, the children can begin to anchor their own sense of safety and security. This restorative work is advocated by Lieberman and van Horn (2004) in their small, but substantive and practical, guide.

Parent–Child Co-Created Narrative Dialogue

I waited purposefully to begin the conjoint work until about 6 months after I began to work with both parent and child individually. Stephanie was feeling much better; had done the rigorous work of trauma processing; and had managed to create a cohesive narrative in which she was able to recall most of the traumatic event, except for the parts mercifully spared by her dissociative episodes and, finally, by her going to sleep (and probably passing out). She had also managed to tell her parents what had happened, and although she had prepared herself for their criticism and rejection, Stephanie's mother confided that she herself had also been raped as a teen but had never spoken about it to anyone. Sharing this intimate information gave Stephanie and her mother an opportunity for closeness and mutual empathy, even though it was fleeting.

In therapy, Stephanie had challenged some of her guilt and shame. As she began to do so, and realized she had not caused the rape (by opening the door or letting the rapist in), the impact of the trauma on her—specifically, her symptoms—began to decrease. One of the indicators of Stephanie's improvement occurred when she chose to break her fear-based secrecy and opted to tell a few choice friends and her pastor about what she had survived. Stephanie reported to me that sharing the secret made her feel "lighter," and that learning directly that nothing bad would come of telling had made her feel empowered. At this stage of recovery, Stephanie was clearer about what she was willing to tolerate from other people, and she continued to grow in confidence and clarity. This newfound confidence was put to the test when the police called her to say that they had apprehended a suspect, and she was asked to come down to the station to see whether she could identify her perpetrator from a lineup. She called to tell me that she was going to the police station and had high hopes that they had found the right person, although she didn't want to get her hopes up.

Stephanie called back to say she was relieved but "shaken up" to see the face of the man she had hoped never to see again. She noted that he looked much smaller and less threatening in the lineup, and that he seemed afraid and uncertain. Stephanie was surprised to have such a range of emotions; she took a long shower and cried when she got home. Stephanie knew that this was just the very beginning of a very long process that she would endure.

Stephanie made great strides in reaching out to friends and rejoining her church activities. She broke her own sense of isolation and stigmatization, and eventually began to feel like her "old self." It was only when she had strengthened her self-image and began to feel more and more competent that I asked her to participate in this work.

Stephanie approached the parent–child sessions with interest but also with apprehension, especially because she knew that she would have to speak about the rape directly to her child and had always felt too paralyzed by her emotions to do so. Allyson, by contrast, actually seemed excited to show her mom around the play therapy office. As a matter of fact, the first session with Stephanie and Allyson was completely nondirective, and Allyson showed her mom everything in the room—even some things she had never played with herself.

In the second session, I told Allyson that she could have some time to do "whatever she wanted" with her mom, but that before she did that, her mom had something that she wanted to talk to her about.

Stephanie was a little nervous, but very ready to have this dialogue with her daughter. She started out by saying, "I know that you remember when that man came into our house and hurt me." Allyson looked at her mom and seemed still. "We've never talked about it because I was hoping that we would both forget what happened. But now I know that it's very hard to forget about it because it was so scary, and I was so hurt that I couldn't help you or hold you."

Allyson rushed to the sand tray miniatures and grabbed the "mean man," bringing it back to her mother. "This is the mean man, Mami; he's the one that hurt you. He's mean." "Yes," Stephanie said, "he was mean and he hurt me a lot, and now he's in jail being punished." Allyson asked, "Why did he hurt you, Mami?" and Stephanie said softly, "I don't know, mija. Some people do not have God in their hearts, and they are mean." Allyson kept talking as if hoping to get in everything she had wanted to say. "I kept coming to your room, Mami, but I was scared and ran away." Stephanie said, "You are a little girl, not a grownup. There was nothing you could do. You are a brave and sweet girl, and there was nothing you could do to help me because the man was strong and bigger than us." "I hate him," Allyson said, throwing the miniature of the mean man on the floor.

This dialogue served as the foundation for five sessions in which Stephanie and Allyson told each other the stories they remembered. As they did, I often paraphrased what they were saying, and when possible I would help organize the narrative by putting the information into a cohesive memory with a beginning, middle, and end. In addition, whenever I had opportunities to incorporate different parts of the memories, I did so. For example, Allyson talked about going back to her room and hiding under the covers. When she described this behavior, I reminded her that she was feeling very scared, that her heart was beating fast, and that she had prayed to God that the man would leave quickly. Such assimilation of memory fragments allows for the co-created narrative to become more and more organized, and for the clients to develop a sense that they are going from a passive role to one of activity—observation, reflection, and understanding.

This conjoint treatment was also critical to enhancing attachment between Allyson and her mother. This attachment had been compromised by the sexual assault, which rendered the mother helpless in her daughter's eyes. Stephanie's role as a protector of her daughter's safety had been gravely compromised, and in order to move forward, Allyson's feelings and needs had to take center stage, in a way they hadn't when her mother was debilitated by her attacker. The last 15 minutes of each of these conjoint sessions included the mother's holding and rocking her daughter, singing to her and comforting her, saying that nothing like that would ever happen again. I remember sitting there hoping that this would be true; I was, and am, sadly aware that life is very unpredictable.

Termination

What is predictable, however, is children's resilience and willingness to reach out over and over. Mother and daughter found solace in the truth and in their ability to have each other as unconditional witness. Mother's ability to provide a context for her daughter to understand what she had seen had been severely compromised by her trauma responses. When Stephanie was able to do her own trauma processing, she was restored to a capable, nurturing figure to her daughter and their speaking together allowed the co-construction of the trauma narrative that included both their perspectives. They were able to be more fully present for each other because they had done their own individual work, in ways that suited them best. Fortification of parents is critical to children's restoration of safety. Children need to know that their parents are capable of protection and guidance. Stephanie was eventually restored to that appropriate and necessary role through parent–child sessions that were trauma focused.

CONCLUDING COMMENTS

This case study clearly illustrates the overwhelming impact of trauma, as well as individual capacities to overcome trauma effects and move forward. At the same time, it indicates the necessity for clinical facilitation utilizing approaches uniquely tailored for traumatized children and adults. The organizing principle is to help individuals face and organize traumatic material that can be experienced in fragmented ways, and can cause havoc with a sense of personal control. While Stephanie was able to participate in talk therapy that included gradual exposure techniques, Allyson had the option of using toys and miniatures to "play out" her trauma experience. The ultimate goal was for this parent–child dyad to bear witness to each other's narrative, clarify questions, identify moments of mastery and help, and develop hope for a safe future.

Stephanie was able to guide Allyson's recovery once she processed her traumatic memories. As mother and child grew stronger independently, they were able to come together, to be connected in their experience in a way that was not possible during the actual event.

My overriding memory is the courage and strength they both accessed and used to reconnect, deal with a historical trauma, and re-engage in their appropriate roles of mother/protector/nurturer and secure and trusting child.

REFERENCES

Axline, V. M. (1969). *Play therapy* (rev. ed.). New York: Ballantine Books.

Booth, P. B., & Jernberg, A. M. (2010). *Theraplay: Helping parents and children build better relationships through attachment-based play.* Hoboken, NJ: Wiley.

DeMaria, M. B., & Cowden, S. T. (1992). The effects of client-centered group play therapy on self-concept. *International Journal of Play Therapy, 1*(1), 53–67.

Dripchak, V. L. (2007). Posttraumatic play: Towards acceptance and resolution. *Journal of Clinical Social Work, 35,* 125–134.

Foa, E. B., & Rothbaum, B. O. (1998). *Treating the trauma of rape: Cognitive-behavioral therapy for PTSD.* New York: Guilford Press.

Gil, E. (2007). Nicolas puts back the pieces: Transforming a childhood trauma. In M. Bussey & J. B. Wise (Eds.), *Trauma transformed: An empowerment response* (pp. 15–35). New York: Columbia University Press.

Gil, E. (Ed.). (2010). *Working with children to heal interpersonal trauma: The power of play.* New York: Guilford Press.

Kot, S. (1996). Intensive play therapy with child witnesses of domestic violence (Doctoral dissertation, University of North Texas, 1995). *Dissertation Abstracts International, 56,* 3002A.

Kot, S., & Tyndall-Lind, A. (2005). Intensive play therapy with child witnesses of domestic violence, In L. A. Reddy, T. M. Files-Hall, & C. E. Schaefer (Eds.), *Empirically based play interventions for children* (pp. 31–49). Washington, DC: American Psychological Association.

Landreth, G. L. (1991). *Play therapy: The art of the relationship.* Muncie, IN: Accelerated Development.

Lieberman, P., & Van Horn, P. (2004). *Don't hit my mommy: A manual for child–parent psychotherapy with young witnesses of family violence.* Washington, DC: Zero to Three.

Marvasti, J. A. (1994). Please hurt me again: Posttraumatic play therapy with an abused child. In T. Kottman & C. Schaefer (Eds.), *Play therapy in action: A casebook for practitioners* (pp. 485–525). Northvale, NJ: Jason Aronson.

Ray, D. (2011). *Advanced play therapy: Essential conditions, knowledge, and skills for child practice.* New York: Routledge.

Schaefer, C. E. (1994). Play therapy for psychic trauma in children, In K. J. O'Connor & C. E. Schaefer (Eds.), *Handbook of play therapy: Vol. 2. Advances and innovations* (pp. 297–318). New York: Wiley.

Shelby, J., & Felix, E. D. (2005). Posttraumatic play therapy: The need for an integrated model of directive and nondirective approaches. In L. A. Reddy, T. M. Files-Hall, & C. Schaefer (Eds.), *Empirically based play interventions for children* (pp. 79–104). Washington, DC: American Psychological Press.

Tyndall-Lind, M. A. (1999). Revictimization of children from violent families: Child-centered theoretical formulation and play therapy treatment implications. *International Journal of Play Therapy, 8*(1), 9–25.

Terr, L. C. (1981). "Forbidden games": Post-traumatic child's play. *Journal of the American Academy of Child Psychiatry, 20*(4), 741–760.

Terr, L. C. (1991). Childhood traumas: An outline and overview. *American Journal of Orthopsychiatry, 148*(1), 1–19.

Chapter 6

Calm, Connection, and Confidence

Using Art Therapy to Enhance Resilience in Traumatized Children

CATHY A. MALCHIODI

According to Siegel (2013), "resilience" can be defined as having flexibility and strength in the face of stress and possessing what is needed to "rise above adversity, learn from experience and move on with vitality and passion" (p. 118). It is strengthened by protective factors such as supportive family members and other caregivers, the capacity for self-regulation, and personal initiative and temperament. However, when children experience crisis or trauma, their capacity for resilience is challenged even if they have support from family and caregivers and a sense of self-efficacy. Although adverse experiences may influence resilience, crisis or trauma may also be opportunities to restore and enhance resilience in children, through strategic interventions that help young clients to develop the skills and relationships necessary to "bounce back."

Art therapy is one approach that provides a child-friendly form of intervention and self-expression to support resilience in young clients. While art therapy is based on the idea that visual expression is a form of nonverbal communication, it is also an action-oriented strategy that can be tailored to complement strength-based goals in treatment. In particular, traumatized children benefit from sensory-based interventions such as art, music, dance/movement, drama, and play therapies as a central part of their recovery process (Malchiodi, 2014a). A recent government document focusing on trauma-informed practices (Substance Abuse and Mental Health Services Administration [SAMHSA], 2014) underscores the importance of adapting arts- and play-based approaches to instill and maintain resilience during the aftermath of both single acute and multiple traumatic events. In trauma-informed care, it is essential to adhere to a strength-based perspective that acknowledges resilience in children, adults, families, and communities in the process of recovery not only from traumatic events themselves, but also from a variety of related psychosocial, cognitive, and physical challenges (SAMHSA, 2014).

This chapter describes how specific art- and play-based interventions can help to enhance and restore resilience in children who have experienced a traumatic event. The general principles of art therapy with children are described, with an emphasis on best practices in applying this approach to support adaptive coping skills, strength-based responses, and secure attachment and connection to caregivers. A case example of a child who experienced a traumatic event is discussed, to illustrate a variety of practical strategies and to help therapists develop their own interventions for enhancing resilience with young clients.

ART THERAPY AND CHILDREN

"Art therapy" can be defined as the application of visual arts and creative processes within a therapeutic relationship, to support, maintain, and improve the psychosocial, physical, cognitive, and spiritual health of individuals of all ages (Malchiodi, 2005, 2012a, 2013). It is part of a larger array of creative arts therapies (art, music, dance/movement, and drama) that emerged as distinct forms of treatment in the mid–20th century. Play therapists, counselors, and psychologists often use art-based approaches with clients, particularly children, to help them communicate feelings and experiences through developmentally appropriate, action-oriented strategies. In fact, art therapy and play therapy approaches often overlap, since each is a creative, action-oriented form of therapy that demands participation and sensory self-expression.

Child art therapy has a long history in mental health treatment, health care, rehabilitation, and education (Malchiodi, 2014b; Rubin, 2005; Shore, 2013). It is often applied in conjunction with various theoretical approaches, including psychoanalytic, object relations, humanistic, cognitive-behavioral, and integrative expressive arts applications (Malchiodi, 2012a). In particular, it is frequently used to address trauma because it allows young clients to express themselves nonverbally. For example, in the aftermath of the terrorist attacks on September 11, 2001, and more recently in interventions with survivors of mass violence such as the 2012 Sandy Hook Elementary School shooting in Connecticut (Loumeau-May, Seibel, Pelicci-Hamilton, & Malchiodi, 2014), art therapy has played a key role in helping children communicate complex reactions to mass trauma. For those who have been abused or violated, art expression is a widely accepted way to communicate feelings and experiences without words. In addition, it is applied in treatment of children with various disorders—including attention-deficit/hyperactivity disorder (Safran, 2012), autism (Gabriels & Gaffey, 2012), and medical illnesses (Beebe, 2013; Council, 2012)—as a form of nonverbal, developmentally appropriate intervention.

Child art therapy often includes art therapy for multiple family members (Kerr, Hoshino, Sutherland, Parashak, & McCarley, 2008; Riley & Malchiodi, 2004) or for parent–child dyads, particularly in attachment work (Malchiodi, 2014a; Proulx, 2009). Art- and play-based approaches are effective ways to introduce social interaction, support interpersonal skills, and encourage positive connections between parents and children because these approaches are often perceived as pleasurable. The sensory nature of art expression also capitalizes on the functioning of the right hemisphere, the area of the brain thought to be responsible for an internal working model for attachment relationships and affect regulation (Schore, 2003; Siegel, 2012). Art therapy is essentially a relational intervention that offers opportunities for connection through active participation, particularly between a parent and child and/or a therapist and young client (Malchiodi, 2014a).

ART THERAPY AND RESILIENCE

Enhancing or restoring resilience has received increased attention in the creative arts therapies as a treatment goal for young clients. For example, research reveals the positive effects of music therapy on coping skills and resilience-related outcomes for patients with pediatric cancer (Robb et al., 2014). Advocates of dance/movement therapy claim that one proven benefit of dancing is an increased sense of vitality that may decrease depression, improve mood, and increase positive feelings about oneself (American Dance Therapy Association, 2014).

Art therapy is noted to specifically promote resilience through collaboration, community, and connection within group settings such as art studios and structured art-making groups; in particular, groups that encourage participation in decision making and empower youth are effective in resilience building (Aumann & Hart, 2009; Macpherson, Hart, & Heaver, 2012). Others observe that it is particularly useful with youth who are at risk for developmental, behavioral, and addiction problems (Stepney, 2009). In general, art-based approaches have been cited as ways to increase quality of life (Madden, Mowry, Gao, Cullen, & Foreman, 2010) and inspire positive emotion (Malchiodi, 2007). With children, art and play therapy strategies are widely employed interventions that support resilience and enhance posttraumatic growth through sensory-based methods (Steele & Malchiodi, 2012), and, as noted above, they capitalize on right-brain-dominant, action-oriented experiences.

In particular, art therapy approaches based on trauma-informed practice include resilience building as a primary goal for children and families. Trauma-informed expressive arts therapy is one model that includes resilience principles in specific applications of art, music, movement, dramatic enactment, play, and imagination (Malchiodi, 2012b, 2014b). In brief, it recognizes that symptoms are adaptive coping strategies rather than pathology, and uses the arts to help individuals move from being "survivors" to "thrivers." This approach is based on the idea that the creative arts therapies are helpful in reconnecting implicit (sensory) and explicit (declarative) memories of trauma and in the treatment of posttraumatic stress disorder (Malchiodi, 2001). It underscores positive connection and attachment, particularly in children who have experienced multiple traumas and losses, and it emphasizes arts-based experiences that reinforce a sense of safety through self-soothing. In brief, a trauma-informed expressive arts therapy approach means providing various opportunities for individuals to engage in creative experimentation that integrates experiences of unconditional appreciation, guidance, and support (experiences found in families that are successful in helping children to flourish). The goal is to help the individuals not only to recover from traumatic experiences, but also to recover the "creative life"—a sense of personal well-being and positive relationships with others.

THE THREE C'S:
CALM, CONNECTION, AND CONFIDENCE

In working with children, I often focus art-based intervention on three specific areas that support and restore resilience: calm, connection, and confidence. "Calm" refers to the basic goal of all treatment, which is to help individuals learn to self-regulate and feel safe while developing skills to reduce stress when faced with upsetting events. "Connection" is the key element in all strength-building intervention; social support and positive attachment are central to resilience throughout the lifespan. "Confidence" involves a sense of mastery that supports an internal locus of control and the belief that one can successfully address challenges. These three areas and related applications of trauma-informed expressive art therapy are explained in more detail throughout the following case example of a child client who experienced an acute traumatic event and whose treatment included a trauma-informed approach capitalizing on resilience-enhancing strategies.

CLINICAL CASE EXAMPLE: KAITLYN

Kaitlyn, a 9-year-old girl, sustained several dog bites while in her backyard. She was playing on a swing set when a large dog running loose in the neighborhood attacked her from behind without provocation. The dog first bit her on her back, dragging her from the swing set for 20 feet while Kaitlyn screamed for help. By the time a neighbor and Kaitlyn's mother reached her, the dog had bitten the child several times on various parts of her body. Another neighbor quickly came to the scene with a gun, and captured and killed the dog within the proximity of Kaitlyn and her mother. A few minutes later, an ambulance, fire truck, and police cars arrived on the scene; Kaitlyn was placed on a stretcher and was rushed by ambulance to a local hospital, along with her mother. The nearest hospital was 15 miles away, making the experience even more tense and frightening for both mother and child. Approximately 30 minutes later, Kaitlyn was admitted to the emergency room for surgery to address her wounds. Despite the seriousness of her multiple dog bites, she was in stable condition by the end of the day and was medicated to address the pain and possibility of infection.

Kaitlyn was expected to make a full recovery, but her wounds required that she remain in the hospital for a couple of weeks. I first saw Kaitlyn on the third day of her stay at the hospital, when I met with her and her mother in her hospital room. Because of the nature of her injuries and medical treatment, Kaitlyn had to remain in a stationary position; at our first meeting, she was propped up by pillows and semirestrained. This was obviously uncomfortable for her because she had previously been a physically active child. She was also fearful of the many medical procedures she was subjected to, even though she understood that the doctors and nurses were trying to help her recover.

Kaitlyn's mother reported that even before the dog bite incident and hospitalization, her daughter had tended to be "shy" and did not seek out support or help from teachers or other adults. She had been told by a counselor at Kaitlyn's school that her daughter was "somewhat overly constrictive" in her behavior and tended to be more withdrawn than hyperactive when stressed. When I asked Kaitlyn's mother how Kaitlyn expressed her feelings when distressed, she said that often her daughter would say simply, "I'm fine," or "I don't know." Kaitlyn's mother added that it seemed that after her divorce, her daughter's communication became more defended, and she could not easily express anger, sadness, or worries. In addition, Kaitlyn often displayed "pleasing behavior," attending to the needs and emotions of her mother or other family members before her own.

Initial Sessions

In my first meeting with Kaitlyn at the hospital, it was obvious that many aspects of her hospitalization, various medical procedures, and her physical restraints were uncomfortable and upsetting. But instead of openly communicating her pain and frustration, Kaitlyn responded to her situation by remaining quiet and withdrawn. I respected her response as an adaptation to an abnormal situation rather than a defense, and allowed Kaitlyn to displace her emotions to something external (e.g., to speak to me through a puppet or cartoon character) rather than to communicate directly about her feelings and experiences. At the same time, in order to enhance Kaitlyn's resilience, I fet that it would also be essential to help her identify how her body responded to stress and worry, strengthen her positive attachment with her mother, and provide experiences of mastery.

In my next session, Kaitlyn was able to engage in some free play with a set of family puppets I brought to her bedside, along with some art materials. As the puppet play progressed, I began asking her whether she could speak for any of the puppets, and if so, what the puppets would say. Kaitlyn puzzled over the request for a few minutes, but then suddenly picked up the girl puppet and said, "She did something very bad . . . 'cuz why would all this bad stuff happen?" She also volunteered that the puppet "always felt crummy because she thought she messed up her mom and dad staying together." When I asked her to tell me a little more about that, she said, "'Cuz this girl did things like burn the waffles in the oven and made a mess in the bathroom. Bad stuff happened to her." Kaitlyn clearly expressed self-blame not only for the dog attack, but also for her parents' divorce. In addition to the stress of hospitalization, she had numerous worries and ruminated about them.

Because Kaitlyn seemed interested in the brightly colored drawing materials I brought to her bedside, I asked her if she would like to draw a picture of any of the puppets. Without hesitation, Kaitlyn took a set of the marking pens and paper and drew an image of her mother, saying, "Mom is the best" (Figure 6.1). From the style and enthusiasm of Kaitlyn's creativity, it was obvious that she loved and admired her mother, depicted her with positivity, and did not blame her mother for not rescuing her from the dog attack.

During the first week of Kaitlyn's hospitalization, I had the opportunity to meet with her mother separately on two occasions. Kaitlyn's mother was understandably distressed by the dog attack, the resulting injuries to her daughter, the subsequent hospital stay, and the probability of many outpatient follow-up visits over several months. I noticed in these meetings with the mother that she tended toward pessimism in her perceptions about herself, noting that "Things just never seemed to work out for me," and "I sometimes believe that I am not lovable" (referring to her divorce from Kaitlyn's father). Like Kaitlyn, the mother lacked confidence and blamed herself for the incident with the dog: "When the dog attacked Kaitlyn, I thought what a terrible mother I must be, a real jerk and failure. I think she must hate me for not being a better parent when this happened." In considering Kaitlyn's puppet play responses, it was clear that both mother and daughter felt responsible for all the "bad stuff" that happened, and that the mother felt like a failure in terms of parenting.

The mother was surprised when I showed her Kaitlyn's drawing of her and relayed Kaitlyn's comment on it (with Kaitlyn's permission); she remarked that she could not believe that her daughter thought she was "the best" mom after the dog attack. Despite this strong perception, Kaitlyn's mother appeared noticeably relieved when presented with the drawing. I remarked that if Kaitlyn was in agreement, they might display the picture in the hospital room (and, after discharge, in a prominent place in the home), where both mother and daughter could see it regularly to serve as a positive reminder of their relationship. This simple illustration is a good example of one of the inherent values of art therapy products: An art expression can serve as a sensory-based, visual reminder that can cue positive responses between sessions.

However, there were many issues to address in regard to Kaitlyn's psychosocial needs, as well as her postinjury and subsequent trauma reactions. The following sections describe a trauma-informed expressive arts therapy approach to support resilience in Kaitlyn and her mother.

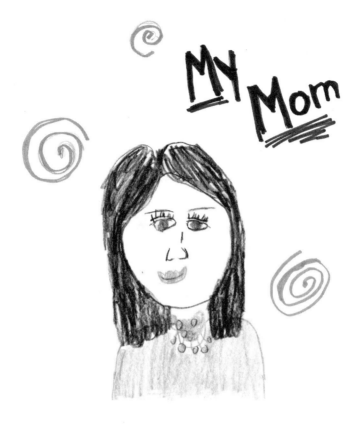

FIGURE 6.1. Kaitlyn's drawing of "My Mom." Reprinted with permission of Cathy A. Malchiodi. Copyright 2014.

In brief, these strategies included enhancing self-regulation and stress reduction; reinforcing positive connection between parent and child; and increasing a sense of mastery through expressive arts and play. Although these three areas of specific intervention are discussed separately, most of the sessions addressed all three goals of treatment (self-regulation, connection, and mastery), with resilience as a core objective.

Calm: Supporting Self-Regulation

"Self-regulation" can be defined as a set of internal skills that includes the abilities to calm oneself when upset and to help oneself feel better despite obstacles and challenges. It also includes the ability to manage experiences on emotional, cognitive, social, and physical levels. Perry (2014) refers to self-regulation as a "core strength" and one that is key to the healthy development of a stress response capability. Whereas some children who are unable to self-regulate are disruptive and labeled "hyperactive," other children (like Kaitlyn) may appear withdrawn, quietly perseverating, and ruminating without relief.

In general, resilient individuals are effective self-regulators; in other words, they are able to remain calm under pressure and to adapt quickly to new challenges. Because self-regulation can be practiced, it is a skill that children can learn to manage stress after traumatic events and to enhance the ability to meet new stressful situations successfully. Art making can be a self-regulating activity in and of itself, if the activity is self-soothing and engaging for the art maker. In other words, the repetitive, sensory-based qualities of specific art-based interventions can help relieve stress and enhance the relaxation response.

Children and their caregivers who are struggling with trauma responses must often be coached in ways to reduce stress and effectively self-regulate in the earliest stages of trauma intervention. A key goal of art therapy with hospitalized children like Kaitlyn is to provide various ways for them to decrease their distress and frustration, and to increase their sense of calm and control. In most hospitals, professionals known as "child life specialists" provide specific self-regulating art and play interventions. In Kaitlyn's case, child life staff members were available to help her understand medical procedures through medical play with syringes, bandages, and other medical toys and props. My role became to offer additional intervention through the use of art and play and related methods of self-regulation; in particular, my goal was to develop strategies that Kaitlyn and her mother could practice at home after the inpatient stay ended. Enlisting parents and other caregivers in supporting self-regulation is central to reinforcing this skill because caregivers play a pivotal role in overall success.

I initially taught Kaitlyn some child-friendly ways to use breathing to calm herself when she felt upset. We practiced "breathing deeply like a sleeping bear," "hissing like a bee," and "roaring like a lion" from our bellies. I also helped Kaitlyn learn how to make a cardboard butterfly that she could balance on the end of her finger when she needed distraction from something upsetting (see Malchiodi, 2014b). Because it was important to include Kaitlyn's mother in some of the sessions, I taught both of them how to make "tangle doodles"—simple marks with colorful felt pens in various familiar and easy designs and patterns, based on a formal method called Zentangle® (Krahula, 2012) that is perceived as an enjoyable, relaxing activity. After Kaitlyn and her mother had a chance to experiment with various designs individually, I introduced the idea of making a joint tangle doodle (Figure 6.2) by tracing their hands

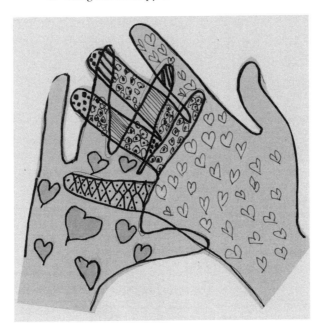

FIGURE 6.2. A mother–daughter "tangle doodle." Reprinted with permission of Cathy A. Malchiodi. Copyright 2014.

overlapping each other on a piece of paper and filling in the spaces with whatever lines and shapes they liked. This not only created another opportunity to engage in relaxing mark making, but also served as a symbolic gesture of connectedness that both parent and child seemed to enjoy.

The experience of tracing her hand inspired another drawing by Kaitlyn in the next individual session with me. She asked me whether she could trace her hand on paper, and then surprised me when she asked to show me how to "draw a dog's face" on the tracing. She carefully and quietly colored the image, asking for a pencil at the end to draw one more part—a chain on the dog's collar (Figure 6.3). When I asked her to tell me about the picture, she quietly said, "Dogs need to be chained 'cuz they can hurt people if they are running around. This dog has a strong chain" (pointing to the chain in the drawing). I did not push her to tell me more about the dog image as related to the specific experience of the dog that hurt her. Instead, I observed, "Sometimes dogs are not chained, and they can roam into other people's yards. But if this happened and the dog hurts someone, it was not the person's fault that she was hurt by the dog. I think it is pretty smart that you thought

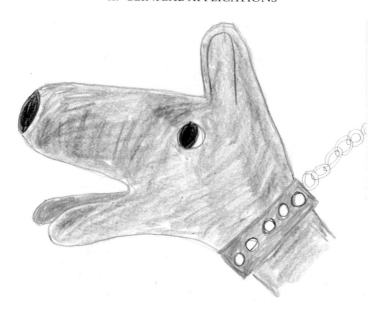

FIGURE 6.3. Kaitlyn's drawing of a "dog's face." Reprinted with permission of Cathy A. Malchiodi. Copyright 2014.

to put a chain on your dog in your drawing." Although it would take many sessions before Kaitlyn really believed that she was not the cause of the dog's attack, she did nod with a slight smile when I highlighted her way of keeping the dog restrained by her imaginary chain.

At this point in therapy, I introduced the concept of "thought catching" from the Penn Prevention Program's "adversity–beliefs–consequences" (ABC) model (Ellis & Dryden, 1987; Seligman, 1995) as an additional self-regulation strategy because both Kaitlyn and her mother tended to engage in self-blame when negative events occurred, automatically perseverating on adversity. In order for both to be able to self-regulate successfully and reduce their stress responses, it was key to help them learn to identify ("catch") thoughts that led to negative feelings and to determine how these emotions felt in the body. I adapted the ABC model process for Kaitlyn and her mother by using simple body outlines, asking them to "catch their worry thoughts" and to show me (through making marks and using colors, shapes, and/or lines) "where the worry is in your body and what it looks like" (see, e.g., Figure 6.4). Over several sessions, this activity helped both child and parent recognize when they were engaging in negative thinking and how to identify

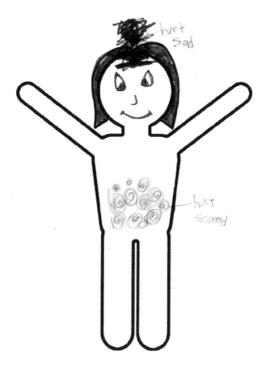

FIGURE 6.4. Kaitlyn's catching of her "worry thoughts" in a body outline. Reprinted with permission of Cathy A. Malchiodi. Copyright 2014.

the associated feelings in their bodies. It thus provided each with the opportunity to apply self-regulation activities to "catch their thoughts" and reduce stress reactions.

Connection: Strengthening Positive Attachment

The presence of a stable, nurturing parent or caregiver is widely accepted as key to instilling and supporting resilience in children. Although Kaitlyn did not feel abandoned by her mother during the dog bite incident, Kaitlyn's mother certainly expressed distress about not having been available quickly enough to stop the dog from harming her daughter. For this reason, both parent and child stood to benefit from sessions focused on strengthening a sense of positive, secure attachment between them. Art and play also became a way for me to model effective communication and activities that Kaitlyn's mother could use with her daughter between sessions and after therapy was terminated.

In art- and play-based activities to support resilience through positive connection, the concept of "attunement" is a key aspect of intervention. Attunement is a relational dynamic that helps build a healthy sense of self in children and is a central feature of every caring relationship and secure attachment (Perry & Szalavitz, 2006; Siegel, 2012). For example, well-attuned caregivers can detect what their children are feeling and experiencing; recognize nonverbal communications; and respond appropriately through verbal, tactile, and other means to reduce children's distress. Good attunement is also related to an experience of "reflexive convergence," in which two people "feel felt" by each other (Siegel, 2012). It promotes flexibility in response to stress, as well as positive attachment—key experiences related to the development of resilience.

There are many ways to apply arts-based interventions to reinforce attunement and reflexive convergence between parents and children. Dyadic art and play therapies in particular are good ways to encourage interaction because parents and children can learn by actively watching and mirroring each other through visual, tactile, movement, rhythm, and auditory senses. For example, a "two-way scribble drawing" is one simple way to structure a dyadic art experience (Malchiodi, 2014a). In this activity, parent and child create a scribble together on one large piece of paper with crayons and felt-tip marking pens or oil pastels. I often make the activity into a game by instructing the parent and child to take turns being the leader in a "scribble chase" across the paper. If the child is the leader, then the parent follows the child's scribble on the paper with a marker or chalk. When the scribble chases are complete, the parent and child can also find shapes or images within the lines and add more colors.

Because Kaitlyn might perceive a "scribble game" as too childish, and she was limited in her range of motion due to her injuries, I developed several creative sessions structured to provide opportunities for dyadic participation in art and play activities focusing on topics relevant to trauma recovery. For example, in one session, the pair was asked to co-create an environment or world in a sand tray for one or two small toy animals (in this case, two rubber ducks) where the animals could feel happy, cared for, and safe. This particular directive was used to open up a conversation between Kaitlyn and her mother about feelings of safety that were compromised by the dog attack and what steps could be put into place for both of them to feel safe in the future if something distressing occurred. It also provided an opportunity to help this dyad reflect on resilience skills they already possessed, but did not recognize.

This session also helped Kaitlyn and her mother them talk about what security, comfort, and nurturance meant to each; for Kaitlyn's mother, this experience helped her identify ways she could be a more effective parent when it came to Kaitlyn's needs for consistent reassurance and validation of feelings.

Finally, strengthening connection between any caregiver and child has more to do with the process itself than with any specific art-based directive to induce positive attachment and enhance resilience. With Kaitlyn and her mother, I introduced many simple but different creative activities that emphasized mutual and reciprocal engagement, and that provided opportunities for both collaborative and parallel art making (individual art making during the same session). Through collaboration, both parent and child strengthened their abilities to resolve problems and develop coping strategies together; in working individually while in sessions together, Kaitlyn and her mother were able to express their personal perspectives to each other. In brief, telling a story about one's art not only validates one's worldview; it also promotes attunement and reflexive convergence through eye contact and verbal and nonverbal communication through creative, playful experiences.

Confidence: Enhancing a Sense of Mastery

"Confidence" actually means many things in terms of enhancing and restoring resilience. It essentially means children's feelings of capability, safety, trust, and positive attachment, despite acute trauma (as in Kaitlyn's case), loss, or multiple adverse experiences. Although self-esteem is often underscored as the key to confidence, it is really a sense of mastery that is most important. Seligman (1995) proposes that whereas self-esteem focuses on feelings associated with strength, more tangible experiences of mastery are the true sources of resilience. Ultimately, the goal of confidence building is to help children perceive themselves accurately, so that when adverse events happen that are not their fault, they will feel competent and worthwhile.

In work with parent–child dyads like Kaitlyn and her mother, a focus on identifying and increasing personal resources for coping with current and future stress or crisis is essential. The Israel Center for the Treatment of Psychotrauma (2014) has developed the "building resilience intervention" (BRI) model, which encourages the development of resilience in children and parents in its ongoing programs with survivors of terrorism and war; it is a useful model that is adaptable to any stressful situation. In the BRI model, children are encouraged to focus on their strengths while expressing their experiences of bombings and life-threatening circumstances. A good example of one of their arts-based resilience-building activities is directing children to invent a device to deal with rocket bombings; children have created depictions of imaginative devices that vacuum up missiles and send them out into space, or invented safe places that can escape the missiles' detection. The goal is to enhance the sensory experience of personal empowerment through active, hands-on participation.

I used a similar approach with Kaitlyn and her mother, helping them to talk about what happened during the dog attack, but at the same time asking them to explore via art materials what they had learned since the attack. Although it is important to provide any traumatized individuals with the opportunity to communicate their memories of and feelings about what happened during the traumatic events, it is equally important to ask them simultaneously to express how the experience may have helped them to become stronger or discover new things. Otherwise, clients are left with only the sensory aspects of the trauma, and do not identify how they have survived and thrived since the crisis or loss occurred. In both joint and individual sessions, Kaitlyn and her mother creatively brainstormed various ideas. In particular, they emphasized their need to develop a plan of action if another unexpected event should ever happen; this eventually became a collage of images for their actual plan of action. The pair bravely included a picture of a swing set, which they decided could be moved closer to the house, where Kaitlyn's mother could see her; they also included a whistle for Kaitlyn to wear to sound a distress signal—or, as Kaitlyn decided, to "scare off animals." Her mother added an image of a church and people; she decided that developing a larger network of social support for herself among members of her church and neighbors would improve her own resilience, thus helping her, as she said, "to be a stronger mom for Kaitlyn."

The point of this and similar art-based activities is to move beyond talk and capitalize on experiencing self-efficacy, personal resources, and coping strategies through the senses. Although we could have simply talked through a plan of action for after termination, action-oriented strategies not only make the hard work of therapy more pleasurable; they also provide positive tactile and kinesthetic experiences that give participants the "felt sense" of mastery. In the case of this mother–daughter dyad, the two created a tangible image that they took home and placed in a prominent spot to serve as a reminder of their plan and the resources they had developed to meet future challenges.

Termination: Recapitulating the Three C's

In our final sessions together, Kaitlyn, her mother, and I had the opportunity to use art and play experiences to recapitulate the resilience goals of the three C's: calm, connection, and confidence. These sessions also provided Kaitlyn with the opportunity to reauthor or reframe the dominant narrative of the trauma story and experience events in new ways (Malchiodi, 2012b). I find that narrative approaches are a good complement to resilience-based work when integrated within overall art and play therapy intervention, and I often use storytelling as a part of the termination process. One particular story that is useful with children who have experienced a life-changing trauma involves the butterfly's life cycle. It draws on the metaphor of a caterpillar changing into a butterfly as a way to demonstrate how things eventually change after a crisis. Butterflies created from cardboard, caterpillar puppets, and a paper bag "cocoon" can be used as props to tell the following story (based on Goffney, 2002). I modified it for Kaitlyn, explaining to her that I wanted to tell her a special story about our work together at the hospital and in outpatient therapy:

> "Do you know where butterflies come from? They start out as eggs and become caterpillars before they become butterflies. Going through a bad experience is like the birth of a butterfly. Before the butterfly is ready to fly free in the world, it has to go through many changes. While all these changes happen, the caterpillar [a prop made from a finger of an old glove] stays safe in its cocoon [I kept the caterpillar in a paper bag].
>
> "When you went through a bad time when the dog attacked you, and then while you were in the hospital, you were very, very brave. Sometimes the only way we can feel better is to stay in our cocoons for a while. While you were in your cocoon, you learned a lot about many different thoughts and feelings. As time went by, you did not need that cocoon as much as you did at first. All of us eventually want to spread our wings and fly again [I made the caterpillar break out of the cocoon and become the butterfly]. Your butterfly learned many new things while in its cocoon, including things it can do to feel better if something upsetting happens."

Although I had a little more of the story to tell, Kaitlyn asked me to stop for a moment so that she could make another butterfly come out of the cocoon. The original butterfly used in the story was part of an activity on self-regulation (balancing a cardboard butterfly on a fingertip); Kaitlyn wanted a second butterfly to emerge from the brown paper bag cocoon. Kaitlyn wrote the word "Mom" on the new butter-fly, to include her parent as a key part of the narrative; we decided to rewrite the story to include both butterflies emerging from their shared cocoon to fly together. In a subsequent termination session with both Kaitlyn and her mother, Kaitlyn enacted her butterfly life cycle and included two butterflies, one for herself and the one she had made for her mother. Although Kaitlyn and her mother still had some challenges to overcome, it was clear that their relationship was strong and that they both had mastered the initial traumatic event that brought Kaitlyn to the hospital.

Finally, during our last session, I strategically presented a children's story called *Shoot for the Moon* (Humphrey, 2011), a tale about a real dog named Rudy who helps his owner learn some important positive lessons about life and resilience. Rudy the dog offers several simple mes-sages about bouncing back from adversity, such as "Don't be afraid of your shadow," "Stretch yourself," and "Just roll with it." One lingering area of mastery that Kaitlyn struggled with involved the understandable fear of dogs. Although she had concluded that the dog who injured her was a "very, very bad dog," Kaitlyn also wanted to have a dog of her own one day. The story of Rudy—whose messages encourage the reader to believe that change is possible—helped Kaitlyn and her mother to have a conversation with me about the future, in which they expressed hope and described strategies for continuing to build confidence and a sense of safety. The story also provided a "virtual therapy dog" for this final therapy session, concluding with Kaitlyn's drawing of "a dog like Rudy" and herself sitting together (Figure 6.5).

CONCLUDING COMMENTS

Kaitlyn and all child trauma survivors can benefit from strategies that identify, enhance, and restore resilience. A trauma-informed approach that includes expressive arts and play is not only developmentally appro-priate for children; it naturally supports active participation from young clients, reinforcing the trauma-informed premises of empowerment and self-efficacy. For Kaitlyn, these included learning ways to self-regulate and reduce stress responses, and developing a sense of mastery through sensory-based, creative activities. For Kaitlyn's mother, a trauma-informed expressive arts approach not only encouraged her co-partici-pation in treatment; it also helped her strengthen a felt sense of her own

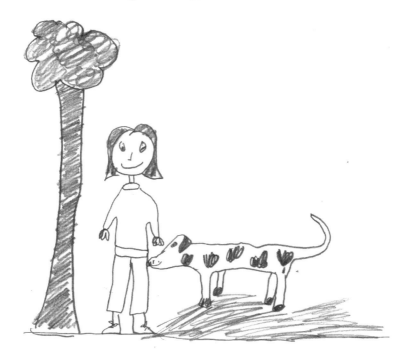

FIGURE 6.5. Kaitlyn's image of herself and "a dog like Rudy." Reprinted with permission of Cathy A. Malchiodi. Copyright 2014.

connection with her child, and allowed her to learn ways to build her own resilience into her parenting.

Art therapy, play therapy, and other creative arts therapies have important roles in any intervention with children who have experienced trauma. Specific and strategic applications of these approaches can support resilience in many ways, but in particular these approaches can be used to provide experiences of self-regulation and stress reduction, positive connection between caregivers and children, and action-oriented experiences of mastery. For Kaitlyn and her mother, art expression served as a way to strengthen their connection as parent and child, reinforce many good memories, and identify coping skills, while still doing the hard work of discussing "what happened" during a frightening and traumatic event. Most importantly, art therapy helps young clients like Kaitlyn actively transform challenges that once seemed hopeless and insurmountable into experiences of self-efficacy through creative means, and thus resume life with greater resilience.

REFERENCES

American Dance Therapy Association. (2014). *Promoting resilience through dance.* Columbia, MD: Author.

Aumann, K., & Hart, A. (2009). *Helping children with complex needs bounce back: Resilient therapy for parents and professionals.* London: Jessica Kingsley.

Beebe, A. (2013). Art therapy with children who have asthma. In C. A. Malchiodi (Ed.), *Art therapy and health care* (pp. 79–91). New York: Guilford Press.

Council, T. (2012). Medical art therapy with children. In C. A. Malchiodi (Ed.), *Handbook of art therapy* (2nd ed., pp. 222–240). New York: Guilford Press.

Ellis, A., & Dryden, W. (1987). *The practice of rational emotive therapy.* New York: Springer.

Gabriels, R., & Gaffey, L. (2012). Art therapy with children on the autism spectrum. In C. A. Malchiodi (Ed.), *Handbook of art therapy* (2nd ed., pp. 205–221). New York: Guilford Press.

Goffney, D. (2002). Seasons of grief: Helping children grow through loss. In J. Loewy & A. Hara (Eds.), *Caring for the caregiver: The use of music and music therapy in grief and trauma* (pp. 54–62). Silver Spring, MD: American Music Therapy Association.

Humphrey, C. (2011). *Shoot for the moon: Lessons on life from a dog named Rudy.* San Francisco: Chronicle Books.

Israel Center for the Treatment of Psychotrauma. (2014). Building resilience intervention (BRI). Retrieved on July 14, 2014, from *www.traumaweb.org/content.asp?PageId=477&lang=En.*

Kerr, C., Hoshino, J., Sutherland, J., Parashak, S. T., & McCarley, L. (2008). *Family art therapy: Foundations of theory and practice.* New York: Routledge.

Krahula, B. (2012). *One Zentangle a day.* Minneapolis, MN: Quarry Books.

Loumeau-May, L. V., Siebel-Nicol, E., Pellicci Hamilton, M., & Malchiodi, C. A. (2014). Art therapy as an intervention for mass terrorism and violence. In C. A. Malchiodi (Ed.), *Creative interventions with traumatized children* (2nd ed., pp. 94–125). New York: Guilford Press.

Macpherson, H., Hart, A., & Heaver, B. (2012). *Building resilience through collaborative community arts practice: A scoping study with disabled young people and those facing mental health complexity.* Brighton, UK: Association for the Help of Retarded Children.

Madden, J. R., Mowry, P., Gao, D., Cullen, P., & Foreman, N. K. (2010). Creative arts therapy improves quality of life for pediatric brain tumor patients. *Journal of Pediatric Oncology Nursing, 27*(3), 133–145.

Malchiodi, C. A. (2001). Using drawings as intervention with traumatized children. *Trauma and Loss: Research and Interventions, 1*(1), 21–27.

Malchiodi, C. A. (2005). *Expressive therapies.* New York: Guilford Press.

Malchiodi, C. A. (2007). *The art therapy sourcebook* (2nd ed.). New York: McGraw-Hill.

Malchiodi, C. A. (2012a). Art therapy and the brain. In C. A. Malchiodi (Ed.), *Handbook of art therapy* (2nd ed., pp. 17–25). New York: Guilford Press.

Malchiodi, C. A. (2012b). Trauma-informed art therapy and sexual abuse. In P. Goodyear-Brown (Ed.), *Handbook of child sexual abuse* (pp. 341–354). Hoboken, NJ: Wiley.

Malchiodi, C. A. (2013). Introduction to art therapy in health care settings. In C. A. Malchiodi (Ed.), *Art therapy and health care* (pp. 1–12). New York: Guilford Press.

Malchiodi, C. A. (2014a). Art therapy, attachment, and parent–child dyads. In C. A. Malchiodi & D. A. Crenshaw (Eds.), *Creative arts and play therapy for attachment problems* (pp. 52–66). New York: Guilford Press.

Malchiodi, C. A. (2014b). Creative arts therapy approaches to attachment issues. In C. A. Malchiodi & D. A. Crenshaw (Eds.), *Creative arts and play therapy for attachment problems* (pp. 3–18). New York: Guilford Press.

Perry, B. D. (2014). Self-regulation: The second core strength. Retrieved on July 3, 2014, from *http://teacher.scholastic.com/professional/bruceperry/self_regulation.htm.*

Perry, B. D., & Szalavitz, M. (2006). *The boy who was raised as a dog.* New York: Basic Books.

Proulx, L. (2009). *Strengthening ties through parent–child dyad art therapy.* London: Jessica Kingsley.

Riley, S., & Malchiodi, C. A. (2004). *Integrative approaches to family art therapy* (2nd ed.). Chicago: Magnolia Street.

Robb, S. L., Burns, D. S., Stegenga, K. A., Haut, P. R., Monahan, P. O., Meza, J., et al. (2014), Randomized clinical trial of therapeutic music video intervention for resilience outcomes in adolescents/young adults undergoing hematopoietic stem cell transplant: A report from the Children's Oncology Group. *Cancer, 120,* 909–917.

Rubin, J. (2005). *Child art therapy.* Hoboken, NJ: Wiley.

Safran, D. S. (2012). An art therapy approach to attention-deficit/hyperactivity disorder. In C. A. Malchiodi (Ed.), *Handbook of art therapy* (2nd ed., pp. 192–203). New York: Guilford Press.

Seligman, M. E. P. (1995). *The optimistic child.* Boston: Houghton Mifflin.

Schore, A. N. (2003). *Affect regulation and the repair of the self.* New York: Norton.

Shore, A. (2013). *The practitioner's guide to child art therapy.* New York: Routledge.

Siegel, D. (2012). *The developing mind: How relationships and the brain interact to shape who we are* (2nd ed.). New York: Guilford Press.

Siegel, D. (2013). *Brainstorm: The power and purpose of the teenage brain.* New York: Tarcher/Penguin.

Steele, W., & Malchiodi, C. A. (2012). *Trauma-informed practices with children and adolescents.* New York: Routledge.

Stepney, S. A. (2009). *Art therapy with students at risk: Fostering resilience and growth through self-expression.* Springfield, IL: Charles C Thomas.

Substance Abuse and Mental Health Services Administration (SAMHSA). (2014). *Trauma-informed care in behavioral health services* (Treatment Improvement Protocol [TIP] Series No. 57, DHHS Publication No. SMA 13-4801). Rockville, MD: Author.

Chapter 7

Utilizing Strength–Based Strategies in the Schools

A School Psychologist's Odyssey

STEVEN BARON

I have been a school psychologist for over a quarter of a century. During that time, the nature of my position has changed dramatically. New mandates, increasing administrative responsibilities, and an emphasis on assessment have gained dominance, at the expense of developing and implementing intervention strategies. One additional phenomenon I have also noted is a tendency of school staff members, who struggle to meet the many mandates now imposed on them, to focus increasingly on students' academic deficits and social shortcomings—as opposed to examining the unique strengths of each pupil.

I became increasingly aware of this neglect of students' strengths during team meetings, Committee on Special Education meetings, and consultations with staff members. Not only does this viewpoint demoralize the staff, but students are likely to be sensitive to this emphasis on deficits as well—and the impact of such thinking on children concerns me greatly. A saying by basketball great Michael Jordan resonates with me: "If you accept the expectations of others, especially negative ones, then you never will change the outcome" (*www.youmotivation.com/ motivational-quotes/22-quotes-by-michael-jordan-4300*). Such negativity not only decreases students' self-esteem, but locks students and teachers into perpetuating this ongoing pattern of low expectations. The overemphasis on negativity thus limits the staff's ability to respond in any alternative manner to the needs of these students, and it promotes a sense of helplessness and bleakness regarding the students' future prospects. I felt myself starting to experience some of these same emotions as this mentality began to infiltrate my own assumptions about how to work effectively with children and staff. It was at this point that I began to reintroduce myself to the field of positive psychology, with its emphasis on a person's attributes as a means to provide support and growth-enhancing experiences. The study of this field has proven to be an effective means of changing my own thinking and ability to work with students, teachers, and parents.

Recent statistics from the Centers for Disease Control and Prevention (CDC) indicate that nearly 20% of children ages 3–17 in the United States have a diagnosable mental health disorder (Ricks, 2013). This rate has been escalating for more than a decade. The geographic region or ethnic background of a child is no shield against the impact of anxiety or depression, with the most common of all maladies, attention-deficit/ hyperactivity disorder (ADHD), affecting nearly 7% of American children. While the emotional cost to children and their families can be devastating, the financial impact on society is overwhelming: The CDC found that the cost of treating diagnosed children is approximately a quarter of a *billion* dollars per year (Ricks, 2013). Approximately 6% of U.S. teens are prescribed medication for a mental health condition (Mann, 2013). As one psychologist recently noted, "this is a very sad growth industry" (Ricks, 2013). As more children are presenting with significant social and/or emotional distress, mental health practitioners will not be the only ones who will need to respond to the unique challenges presented by these children: School personnel will also need to have access to the appropriate methodology to assist both children and their families and mental health care providers effectively.

THE VULNERABILITIES OF STUDENTS

Schooling in the early 21st century is a vastly different experience than in previous times. Educators and students are presented with obstacles that were previously absent or have become much more prevalent. Some of the most pressing issues include the following:

• *Poverty.* In the United States, the poverty rate (more than 15%) is the highest it has been since the 1960s, according to the U.S. Census. The number of school-age children affected by poverty exceeds 13 million (Hayes, 2013). The American Psychological Association reports that the dropout rate for teenagers living in poverty is 10 times higher than for their more affluent peers (Rumberger, 2013).

• *Curriculum changes.* Across the United States, efforts are being made to help students make up deficits in their academic achievement as compared to that of their counterparts in other nations. Not only has this led to debate about the kind of subjects to be emphasized (e.g., science and math at the expense of the humanities), but teaching methodologies are changing, with new types of course syllabi being introduced that require new types of reasoning. This has led to the implementation of extensive assessment programs not only to evaluate students' understanding of material, but to assess teachers' performance. In response, parents and educators alike have raised questions about the excessive pressure this places on all participants.

• *Violence.* Acts of aggression against students and school staff, ranging from bullying to school shootings, are becoming more widespread. A disturbing percentage of students have reported that they are more afraid of harm or attack at school than away from school (U.S. Department of Education, National Center for Education Statistics, 2013).

• *Funding difficulties.* Money for funding public schools continues to be a topic of volatile political debate. School districts are cutting staff and programs to help reel in spiraling costs, as well as to cope with decreasing government funding. These cuts limit all aspects of school functioning: They hinder districts' efforts at recruiting high-quality teachers, reducing classroom size, maintaining after-school programs, purchasing new textbooks, implementing new technologies, providing high-quality support services to students and families, and building new schools.

It is against this contemporary backdrop of challenges that students, parents, and educators must band together on a daily basis. Although working to achieve student success both in academic and social domains is a demanding task for all under these circumstances, this task becomes even more complicated when students present with vulnerabilities. All students are entitled to the best that schools can provide, but school personnel are discouraged by the previously cited challenges. Research suggests that some educators prefer teaching pupils with physical or intellectual limitations to working with children with social, emotional, or behavioral issues (Avramidis & Norwich, 2002). Schools themselves may constitute a risk factor for some students who experience academic frustration and social isolation; their experiences in school may actually exacerbate their presenting issues. Contrarily, a positive school experience can help protect vulnerable children by giving them the tools—and, most importantly, the self-confidence—to flourish, despite the presence of very daunting odds. School psychologists and other counselors must have at their disposal methodologies not only to help students become the best they can be, but to also to address the impact of the above-described factors on staff members' morale and effectiveness.

POSITIVE PSYCHOLOGY

The perspective discussed in this chapter is a strength-based orientation known as "positive psychology." This approach has been developed and championed by many prominent psychologists, including Martin Seligman, Ann Masten, and Michael Rutter, as well as the three editors of this volume. It is defined on the home page of the Positive Psychology Center website at the University of Pennsylvania (*www.ppc.sas.upenn. edu*) as follows: "Positive Psychology is the scientific study of the virtues that enable individuals to thrive. The field is founded on the belief that people want to lead meaningful and fulfilling lives, to cultivate what is best within themselves and enhance their experiences of love, work, and play."

In other words, a strength-based perspective focuses on the development of capabilities and competencies within children and adults, to help them solve problems and live their lives in a more effective manner. It is very important to note that the strength-based orientation does not minimize the pain a person experiences; in fact, it acknowledges the importance of fully understanding it, so as to help create effective interventions. To quote the subtitle of a recent book edited by David A. Crenshaw, a goal of this approach is "honoring strengths without trivializing suffering" (Crenshaw, 2010).

This strength-based view is relatively new, compared to the traditional psychological perspective, which has emphasized pathology as an expression of the traditional medical model. The strength-based model is not so much a series of techniques as a personal perspective that can have a significant impact on how individuals process life events, as well as how they view themselves. It constitutes a holistic approach to working with children in particular: It does not focus on "fixing deficits" within children, but instead on helping the children become more attuned to their strengths and on utilizing these strengths in the healing process. Helping children to discover or reconnect with their assets promotes the children's ownership of what they have previously accomplished and plan to accomplish in the future.

A major component of the strength-based model is "resilience" in children. Although resilience is related to inborn temperament, it can also be enhanced by significant adults in a child's life, such as parents, teachers, coaches, and others. Such adults have been labeled by psychologist Julius Segal as "charismatic adults"—that is, figures who can help children gather strength by helping the children feel special while not denying their difficulties (Brooks & Goldstein, 2001, 2002, and Chapter 1, this volume). The quality of resilience as fostered by such adults can be described as

> the ability of a child to deal more effectively with stress and pressure, to cope with everyday challenges, to bounce back from disappointments, adversity, and trauma, to develop clear and realistic goals, to solve problems, to relate comfortably with others and to treat oneself and others with respect. . . . Resilience explains why some children overcome overwhelming obstacles . . . while others become victims of their early experiences and environments. (Brooks & Goldstein, 2001, p. 1)

Resilience is not limited to the intellectually gifted or most talented people in the general population. Indeed, it is far more common than we might expect. In a classic paper on this subject, Masten (2001) concludes:

> Resilience does not come from rare and special qualities, but from the everyday magic of ordinary, normative human resources in the minds, brains, and bodies of children in their families and relationships, and in their communities. . . . The conclusion that resilience emerges from ordinary processes offers a far more optimistic outlook for action than the idea that rare and extraordinary processes are involved. (p. 235)

This conclusion has far-reaching implications for the development of societal programs and clinical interventions. Such programs and interventions can foster strategies for facilitating the development of adaptive processes within specific children, and can also be applied to specific environments. In particular, schools provide vast opportunities to help children develop and put into practice strengths that might have previously been overlooked. Not only do schools provide the opportunities for students to meet academic goals, but they offer many contexts for the building of adaptive relationships with peers and adults.

Although schools can indeed provide many challenges to students in both the academic and social spheres, they can also provide opportunities for children to learn that prior maladaptive modes of responding to adversity are not their only options. With the support of a caring, supportive staff, students can begin to experience themselves as having the means not only to improve their immediate situations, but also to broaden their self-perceptions as they gain in self-confidence. Methodology based in research on resilience can help children view themselves as being active participants in negotiating complex environmental demands, rather than as ineffective in dealing with concrete problems.

Students spend an average of approximately 32.5 hours a week in school (Swanbrow, 2004), which translates into nearly 1,300 hours over the course of a single academic year. That considerable period of time can be used to increase children's sense of their own competence. In fact, school personnel may indeed have greater opportunities to promote the development of competence within children than parents do, as a recent survey reveals that a typical working parent spends only 19 minutes a day on average interacting with a child to the exclusion of other activities ("19 Minutes," 2014).

One reason why the strength-based approach resonates with me is that school psychologists are often called on to formally assess students' eligibility for classification as having potential disabilities. As I and other members of my school-based support team assessed increasing numbers of students within our domains, we found ourselves paying more attention to spotlighting the extent of the students' weaknesses. This would then lead to a series of meetings in which parents, teachers, and members of the evaluation team would focus on the students' deficits. Invariably, the topic of how to remediate identified weaknesses dominated all discussions. Although these are all very important points in understanding such students, this created a mindset of spotlighting potential failure and remediation, rather than building on the assets in the students' academic and social portfolios.

As these discussions of deficits continued, I became increasingly aware of the ways in which they were affecting all of us. We began to view ourselves as being problem identifiers and fixers, rather than being able to serve in a proactive role to identify and utilize a students' assets that were being overlooked. In addition, we felt that we ourselves were not making full use of all our skills, and this had further adverse effects on our morale. Masten, Herbers, Cutuli, and Lafavor (2008) have made the cogent point that it is crucial to consider the resilience of the adults who work in a school, as these people will play a critical role in fostering a sense of overall school resilience. A resilience-building perspective offers school staff members various opportunities to serve as models of strength for students, enhancing their sense of professional satisfaction.

Another feature of the strength-based perspective is that it can be applied to various populations. Rather than being limited to victims of trauma and other crises, positive psychology and the resilience-building strategies that emanate from it can be applied to a much broader population (Brooks & Goldstein, 2001). In other words, not only can a positive psychology framework be implemented as a reactive measure to trauma, but proactive methods can and should be developed to strengthen adaptive processes for all (Goldstein & Brooks, 2013). Thus students do not have to be formally identified as having weaknesses or disabilities to benefit from strength-based interventions. This perspective allows us to move beyond a reactive or reparative stance and make available to all children the opportunities to become increasingly competent and optimistic, and to develop effective problem-solving and coping skills. In a school environment, the strength-based model can be applied in a variety of contexts—with students on an individual basis or within a classroom, as well with parents and staff.

THE APPLICATION
OF A STRENGTH-BASED APPROACH

I decided to apply some of these principles in my clinical work with students, parents, and staff. As I did, I discovered that participants were often very willing and highly motivated to implement these ideas, and this motivation helped ensure their participation. Also, as participants began to see success, it further increased their commitment to considering and applying the suggestions that were offered. As teachers experienced their students responding constructively to the new ideas, they would often attempt to extend these strategies to other students as appropriate. A further advantage of the strength-based framework is that the interventions typically do not have a major impact on budgetary considerations, since they cost little if anything to implement and are not particularly difficult to set up. For the staff members who participated, their openness to attempting some of these suggestions changed their perspectives about particular children; just as importantly (if not more so), children experienced a shift in their own beliefs about themselves.

The strength-based approach is not an assortment of rote techniques; rather, the methods employed flow from utilizing the strengths and assets of each child in as natural a manner as possible. This ideology lends itself to the application of concrete and easy-to-implement methods, as well as providing a framework to use in counseling sessions with students and in school-based meetings. What follows is a collection of vignettes illustrating various applications of the strength-based model, along with a consideration of how the basic principles of positive psychology guided the development of the specific interventions described. To protect the confidentiality of students and others, identifying data have been altered, but the essence of the strategies and concepts remains intact.

Clinical Case Example: Mary

Mary was a third grader who arrived late for school each morning, resisting efforts by her mother to get her there on time. Mary told her mother on a daily basis that she "hated" school—a setting in which she did not participate in lessons, often kept her head on her desk, and ignored peers. (She was taking medication to address issues with attention.) Mary's highly negative attitude toward school contributed to her avoidant behaviors.

I consulted with Mary's teacher, and we brainstormed how we could provide Mary with a reason to attend school and arrive on time. We came upon the idea of offering Mary a classroom job that would intrigue her enough to do this. I suggested assigning Mary the position of "attendance monitor." The teacher had pointed out that Mary enjoyed being in charge of activities and demonstrated a capacity for organization. The idea of her being responsible for this important job would tap into this ability. I suggested that Mary be given a clipboard to record the daily attendance, to reinforce to her that she indeed had an "official" job.

When we discussed this idea with Mary's mother, she indicated that Mary's behavior at home was very contrary. Although the mother loved the idea of her daughter's having this special job, she was very concerned about her home behavior. I suggested a "Good Behavior" book for home use: Mary's parents would keep a daily list of prosocial behaviors that Mary engaged in (no matter how big or small they might have been), and at the end of the day when the parents were putting Mary to bed, the list would be reviewed with her. (I originally learned about this idea from Paris Goodyear-Brown [2012], a noted play therapist.) Mary's mother agreed to do this.

Follow-up with the teacher indicated that Mary immediately accepted her classroom job; within a few days her affect became increasingly animated and happy, and she began interacting more frequently with peers. She also began arriving at school on time, very eager to perform her job, which seemed to set a positive tone for the rest of the school day. Mary's mother shared that there had been a marked improvement in Mary's behavior at home as well. Mary enjoyed talking about being the attendance monitor, and also took great pleasure in reviewing her daily accomplishments with her parents, which further enhanced their relationship.

In this case, the interventions used by Mary's teacher and mother helped to change Mary's experience at both school and home from significant levels of frustration and disappointment, to feeling recognized for having something meaningful to contribute. Mary's teacher did not present being an attendance monitor as being a necessary chore to complete, but rather as a request for Mary to help out and contribute. I felt that the teacher was explicitly communicating to Mary that she could be a valued member of the class with something to offer, while also instilling a sense of responsibility. From this vantage point, it is not surprising that Mary responded immediately and positively. In addition, Mary found the task to be fun, which was self-reinforcing.

Clinical Case Example: Ralph

Ralph was a 12-year-old boy who had been diagnosed as being on the autism spectrum. He was quick to lose his temper when he became frustrated, particularly by academic requirements. One day his teacher escorted Ralph to my office, as he was very agitated and had just had a tantrum in class. I waited until he calmed down, and then I asked him what happened. He told me that while working on an arts and crafts project, he had made a mistake and could not change it. He began to get upset while describing what happened, and then sat silently.

As I listened to Ralph, I began trying to formulate a response within a strength-based framework that would be meaningful for him. I decided to try something a bit out of the ordinary: I took out a pencil and held it in front of him. I asked him what this was, and he laughed (which in itself was a positive change from how he was feeling and behaving when he came to see me). When he correctly responded, I then asked what the thing on the top of the pencil was called, and he correctly responded, "An eraser." He gave me a quizzical look, and I said, "Pencils have erasers because people are expected to make mistakes. That is part of learning anything new."

Ralph began to cry, saying that he was "horrible" in art. I then asked how hard he had tried on his current project, and, as I expected, he said he had indeed tried very hard. I pointed out to him that the effort he'd put into his project should not be forgotten. As long as he tried—and, in this case, he had tried very hard—he could always be proud. At this point, Ralph reminded me that I had previously told him about Willie Stargell, a great professional baseball player, who amassed a high number of hits during his career but also accumulated a large number of strikeouts. What I had previously told him was that Stargell had once said he became such a proficient hitter by learning so much from striking out. Thus he attributed his success in large part to his failures (Stargell, 1983).

When Ralph reminded me of this, I have to admit that I was surprised. I told him how impressive it was that he had remembered the Stargell story. He then laughed and said that even with the mistake he'd made, he was still going to take the drawing home to his mother to show her, since he had originally intended it for her. I shared with him that not only would this make his mother happy, but it was nice to see that he was not letting what happened hold him down.

The next day, Ralph arrived at my office and explained that he wanted to show me a PowerPoint presentation he had created the previous evening (a few hours after he was brought to my office) for a class assignment. I was impressed by the quality of what he had created. This was a strength of his that I had not been aware of, and we talked about not only what he showed me, but how he became so proficient in designing PowerPoint presentations. Ralph took obvious delight in sharing his work with me. As our time together that day came to a close, I told him that I was very happy he had shared all this with me, and added that making mistakes is sometimes necessary to get us to where we want to be. He looked at me and said, "I see that from yesterday." This was indeed a very touching moment for both of us.

In this instance, I felt that the first interaction with Ralph helped to set the stage for his completing the subsequent assignment and wanting to share it with me. Ralph experienced himself as failing when he felt he did not measure up to his own or others' expectations. The purpose of my comments to him was to help Ralph experience mistakes not as setbacks, but rather as opportunities to learn and benefit from. This is a crucial dimension of a resilient mindset: accepting that mistakes occur and are not the end of the world. The fact that Ralph was able to go home that evening and work on creating an impressive PowerPoint presentation demonstrated that he had understood this. Although much further work in this domain was necessary, it was an important first step that allowed him to take another risk. Ralph's experiencing a mistake as an event to learn from it sent the message that change is indeed possible. It was apparent not only that the message conveyed to Ralph resonated with him, but that he felt accepted, as seen in his wanting to show me the later assignment he had completed.

Clinical Case Example: Fred

Fred was a fourth grader who, like Ralph, was diagnosed as being on the autism spectrum. Although Fred was very bright, he had a great deal of difficulty adapting to changes in routine and to new projects or demands placed upon him. His class had begun preparing to put on a show for parents and students. As part of the show, each student would receive a short solo piece to sing, in addition to participating in a dance with classmates. During rehearsals, the teacher had approached me to voice her concerns over Fred's being able to participate, as he had significant difficulty remaining still while on stage. The teacher asked me how she could remove Fred from the show without upsetting him and his parents.

It was apparent that this teacher's mindset was that Fred would embarrass both himself and the teacher by not being able to behave appropriately. I reminded the teacher that Fred had indeed learned his lines quickly, and also that he had appeared in the previous year's show without any difficulty. At that point, I followed up with Fred and designed a contract with him specifying the behaviors he needed to demonstrate. Before rehearsals, either I or the assistant teacher in the class would review the contract with him. Fred initially showed an improvement in his behavior, but as the date of the show drew closer, he again began to demonstrate disruptive behaviors. I spoke to Fred about this, and he made it clear that he very much wanted to be part of the show.

The teacher was now insisting that Fred be banned from the show. In response, I listed all of his assets, especially his high level of motivation to participate. I made the point that while he would need redirection at times, we should not overreact; we should encourage him to succeed, instead of focusing primarily on his off-task behaviors. The teacher reluctantly accepted this and allowed him to remain in the show (although I certainly had the feeling that if things did not go well, she was going to hold me accountable).

On the day of the show, after some initial moments of Fred's being "antsy" on stage and being briefly redirected by the teacher, he settled in—and, in her words, he was "perfect." Fred's father subsequently contacted me to report that 2 days before the show, Fred had designed his own behavior chart and was very excited that he was able to live up to the goals he put down, which to a large extent mirrored the original chart we had constructed together. I reflected to Fred's father that by nurturing his enthusiasm and providing support, the parents and I had helped to give Fred an incentive to succeed. Fred's father ended our conversation by sharing that not only were he and his wife very proud of Fred, but Fred was also extremely pleased with himself.

This vignette illustrates several points. First, as educators, we should not be too quick to "throw in the towel" on a particular child—especially when there is evidence to suggest that the child's natural talents and skills can indeed be applied to the situation. In this case, I felt that not only did I have to assist Fred in becoming more sensitized to his own behaviors and their possible impact on his goal of wanting to be part of the show, but the teacher's mindset had to be addressed as well. The assumptions we hold about students and colleagues will certainly affect our work and behavior. In this instance, the teacher's negative script about Fred affected her attitude toward him and increased her frustration level with him. My reminding this teacher of Fred's numerous assets helped her acknowledge, although initially grudgingly, that Fred did have something to offer and should be allowed to share it. Gradually the teacher took a more active role in supporting Fred in his quest to perform. The teacher's change in mindset thus contributed to Fred's success in the show. To expect Fred to be the sole party who had to change was both unfair and unrealistic. The teacher's attitude toward Fred began to change when she was finally able to be less reactive and angry toward him and to support him more actively.

In addition, I felt that this experience helped me relate to Fred in a new way. Prior to this, I experienced Fred as being distant and difficult to connect with, which in retrospect I may have been too quick to attribute to his being on the autism spectrum. Seeing how well he responded to a strength-based perspective changed my own reactions to and perceptions of Fred. I soon noticed that my interactions with him following the show changed: Fred was now increasingly verbal with me, and in fact shared that he enjoyed speaking with me. I have noticed with other children as well that after they experience success or feel validated, they often relate in a more open manner in counseling sessions or in other interactions I have with them. Working within a strength-based model promotes a more positive way of relating between children and adults.

Clinical Case Example: Maria

Maria, a 14-year-old female, was self-referred to me. This girl's life circumstances were incredibly sad and overwhelming. Both of her parents had very debilitating illnesses, and her sibling had a profound developmental disability. Her teachers and her parents shared that Maria was extremely depressed, as she often cried and said, "I hate my life." Despite these circumstances, her teachers all reported that they "loved" Maria, as she was hard-working, extremely pleasant, and academically successful.

In the first session, Maria was like a dam ready to burst. She could not wait to launch into the circumstances of her life, especially the impact on her of her parents' illnesses. In addition, Maria had very recently had disagreements with two of her closest friends, and she now feared she was losing a vital support system. Her sobs filled the room. I gave her a few minutes to compose herself, and then I asked about her relationships with these friends. My purpose in doing so was not necessarily to get more details about the conflict, but instead to have her talk about the time she felt closer to these friends and what that was like for her. I also was curious about what might have changed not only about her friends, but about her.

Maria thought about my questions, and she replied that her father's illness in particular had become increasingly worse over the past few weeks and this was a major stressor for her. I then asked whether this could be changing how she was relating to her friends. She sat quietly for a few moments before saying that she might have become more irritable and less patient with others during this time. I pointed out how these feelings were indeed understandable, given what she was experiencing. I then described how her teachers saw her: as someone with numerous strengths and resources, including her strong work ethic, her consistently high level of achievement, and her very positive manner of relating to peers and adults in general. She smiled and said that this really meant a lot to her. I responded that although the circumstances she was dealing with were real and difficult, they were not things she could control. I told her that things she could control were how she worked in school and how she related to other people. She could continue to support her family, but at the same time should not neglect her own needs. Perhaps she could begin to consider what dimensions of her life she could influence and could begin to address. At this point her body relaxed, and she said that she would like to continue this discussion in subsequent sessions, as time had run out.

Several points are highlighted in this example. Throughout my meeting with Maria, I felt I had to walk a fine line between respecting her suffering and honoring her strengths. I certainly tried to validate and empathize with Maria's acutely sad and difficult situation, while at the same time attempting to convey the message that while she had no control over her parents' illnesses, she could direct her responses to these circumstances. I tried to help Maria begin to understand the concept of personal control—another characteristic of a resilient mindset (Brooks, 2003). My goals were to help Maria consider this notion so that she could begin to examine how she was handling this situation, and to empower her to change those aspects of it that were within her influence.

In Maria's case, there was little likelihood of her life circumstances' changing, which served to reinforce her sense of despair and hopelessness. However, rather than continuing to feel helpless in the face of such daunting circumstances, she could strive to have an impact on those parts of her life that could be modified. This would promote a mindset allowing Maria to assume an increased degree of ownership over her life. In fact, research confirms that the greater the degree of personal control people perceive having over their circumstances, the more improvement they demonstrate in both their physical and mental health (Brooks, 2003). The other aim of my meeting with Maria was to help her explore the possibility that her current responses to her life situation, while understandable, might have been having a negative impact on her relationships with others. As she had a long history of positive relationships with others, our discussion helped her to understand that indeed her recent attitudes and behavior might have been affecting her friendships.

Clinical Case Example: Mr. Green

A helpful feature of the strength-based approach particularly in a school setting is that it can be applied in a consultation model with school staff members, thus influencing students in an indirect yet valuable manner. The case of Mr. Green, a middle school teacher, illustrates this point. Mr. Green had sought me out to discuss his concerns regarding a student in his class. Mr. Green reported that this student was exhibiting extremely low functioning in several academic areas; even when it appeared that progress was being made, these hopes were dashed, as there was very little carryover to new situations.

Mr. Green's affect became increasingly depressed as he stated that he was feeling very inadequate as a teacher because of the minimal gains this student was making. He had concluded that this student did not belong in a mainstream class and should be evaluated for a more restrictive setting. Although there might have been some merit to Mr. Green's suggestion for placement of this student, it was clear that his mindset had begun to decrease his confidence about working effectively with this student. In listening to Mr. Green, I decided that it could be useful to address this mindset, but in a manner that he would not perceive as critical. I replied to him that if the strategies and ideas he implemented were not yielding the level of success he had hoped for, he could view the lack of success as an opportunity for him to "think outside the box" and experiment with novel approaches to reaching this student. For example, as a change of pace, he could hold a lesson in the schoolyard with materials found outside, to illustrate concepts that this student was currently working on (botany). I suggested that he had nothing to lose in trying a different approach, and that this suggestion was just one possible idea. At this point, I noticed a marked change in Mr. Green's affect: He seemed to perk up and began to brainstorm about other possible approaches. I went on to add that if he really felt this child belonged in a more restrictive setting, he could ask the special education teacher who worked with students he felt were similar to his student for additional ideas.

In the preceding scenario, I did not view myself as being responsible for offering a ready-to-use suggestion to change this situation. Although I did make one proposal, it was important for me to respect the skills and professionalism of my colleague, who (as I already knew) was an excellent teacher. I felt that his negative mindset about his competency was creating a stalemate in his work with this pupil. Once he began to accept that he could indeed have the freedom to change or modify his approach with this student, it seemed to free up his thinking as he began to consider different possibilities.

This vignette highlights the importance of personal control. A sense of helplessness permeated Mr. Green's self-perception as a teacher. When he began to realize that even in this situation with a challenging student, there were still dimensions that he could indeed control, it stimulated his thinking and inherent creativity. It also served to change his inner dialogue or script about the situation: It allowed him to focus on what he could do, rather than either waiting for the student to change somehow on his own or seeking a change in the student's placement.

Because personal control is a significant feature of a resilient mindset, it is important to for us to recognize that if our efforts with certain children over a period of time have not worked, then it is time for us to consider changing our scripts rather than continuing to wait for the children to change theirs (Brooks & Goldstein, 2001). In this case, it was important for Mr. Green to see that considering alternative solutions to the problem was not "giving in" to a difficult student, but rather a means of empowerment for him as an educator. Furthermore, it is worth considering that the student might consciously or unconsciously have recognized Mr. Green's initial negative mindset, and that this recognition could have played a part in fueling the difficulties he was experiencing.

Clinical Case Example: Michael

The mother of 12-year-old Michael, another boy who was diagnosed as being on the autism spectrum, contacted me to request a meeting to discuss a particular difficulty her son was having. When I met with Michael's mother, she shared that when there was a fire drill at school, her son would refuse to leave the classroom to accompany the rest of the class to the schoolyard. The latest occurrence of this had resulted in the school's suspending her son for a couple of days, and Michael's mother felt this was an unfair punishment.

I asked whether Michael could join us, so I could learn more about the facts of this case. When Michael entered my office, I asked him if he could explain what happened. He calmly told me that the very loud bells, in combination with being surrounded by so many other children, were very frightening to him. Michael's mother added that this had been a difficulty for several years. Michael's mother argued further that suspending him was not really a punishment for Michael, since he was not fond of school.

As Michael described his feelings during fire drills, it was evident that he was experiencing a significant degree of anxiety in reaction to being overstimulated. Michael's mother asked for any intercession or other assistance I could offer in this situation; her own prior conversations with school officials had not been successful in reaching a solution. I began to think of a resolution to this situation that would in the long run meet the school's needs to maintain the health and safety of each student, while respecting Michael's emotional reactions during fire drills. I knew Michael to be very bright, and in fact he had been very expressive in sharing his reactions during this meeting. At that point, I suggested that Michael could write an essay explaining in detail his emotional reactions during a fire drill. He could present it to the school principal, and it would serve as a starting point for discussing possible solutions to this long-standing problem. Michael and his mother reacted very positively to this suggestion, and Michael wrote an essay that he handed in to the school principal. As a result, the suspension was canceled. Michael, his mother, and the principal also had a discussion of Michael's reactions and were able to formulate a compromise solution for future fire drills.

In meeting with Michael and his mother, I felt that my first goal was to convey to both of them that they were being heard in an empathic manner. Michael's mother had entered the meeting feeling very angry, and my first goal was to help her see me (in my role as psychologist) as not being similar to the administrators she had previously dealt with. And allowing Michael the opportunity to share his feelings communicated to both of them that I was taking their concerns seriously. Although I was not in a position to provide a definitive solution, I wanted to utilize Michael's strong ability to express himself as a catalyst for further discussion with the school administration in an antagonism-free manner.

Michael enjoyed expressing his feelings in his essay and again with the principal, who was open to what Michael was saying. In this case, therefore, utilizing an asset of Michael's began a constructive dialogue that served to lessen any ill feelings Michael and his mother had toward the school. Michael learned that appropriate self-expression could be very helpful in resolving disagreements. Furthermore, Michael's essay and the subsequent discussion enabled the school staff to understand Michael better and to see him not as overly contrary or resistant, but as a child whose needs were genuine and required to be met in a different manner.

Clinical Case Example: Dawn

One of my duties as a school psychologist is to chair Committee on Special Education (CSE) meetings, which determine initial or continued eligibility of students for special education services. In this particular instance, I was chairing a CSE meeting regarding a third- grade girl named Dawn, who presented with a significant reading difficulty that contributed to her shutting down to avoid doing work that caused her much frustration. Her teachers were very bothered by her response. As the meeting began, I had Dawn's mother talk about her concerns; and as she listed them, I could feel the "vibe" in the room turn increasingly sad. The special education teacher and classroom teacher each validated Dawn's difficulties. An air of helplessness and hopelessness filled the room.

Finally I asked Dawn's mother, "What do you see as your daughter's strengths? What part of her personality is captivating for you?" In retrospect, I am not sure why I used the word "captivating"; perhaps it was my reaction to the somberness that filled the room. In any case, it did have the effect of altering the mood of the meeting. Dawn's mother thought for a few moments and replied, "She is a good girl. She is just so frustrated." After a pause she went on to say, "She really likes art." I asked her to elaborate on this, and she reported that Dawn loved to draw and was in fact very talented at it. Her teachers had no idea about this. I then asked the teachers whether perhaps her love of art could be incorporated into learning activities. For instance, I said that instead of reading about George Washington, maybe Dawn could draw a picture of him and describe some interesting facts about him.

At this point, the two teachers began to strategize about how they could utilize Dawn's talent for art. In just a few minutes, the tone of the meeting went from despair to invigoration and enthusiasm. Other staff members present suggested that Dawn enter local art contests, and when I asked about art lessons, Dawn's mother replied that she was already considering enrolling Dawn in these. After the meeting, one of the staff members who participated told me how she really liked the question I asked about Dawn's "captivating" qualities, as she could feel the palpable shift in the mood of the meeting at that point. I remember thinking as I left the room that the meeting ended up being just as uplifting for the staff members as it was for the parent.

In fact, this *was* a very powerful meeting for all participants. A fundamental change in the mindset of all who took part occurred. When teachers (or, for that matter, anyone) feel exceedingly negative about a situation, they do not readily envision any change as possible. Asking the question about Dawn's strengths required all those present to change their thinking about her. In short, this line of questioning helped everyone to identify this student's "islands of competence"—a term coined by Brooks for a person's areas of potential success. Brooks and Goldstein (2002) explain:

> If children do not believe they are competent in any arena they are likely to feel insecure and vulnerable. . . . We must remember that an important feature of the resilient mindset is the belief that we all have strengths. Success breeds success. Identifying and reinforcing one island of competence can serve as the catalyst to attempt other challenges. (p. 158)

Attempting to identify Dawn's "islands of competence" was what happened in the meeting. As Dawn's teachers were able to break free of their previous ideas about Dawn, they were able to brainstorm and feel empowered as educators. When anyone is feeling stuck, it is not uncommon to hold an external party responsible for the predicament. Blaming does not lend itself to change, as it gives the locus of control to someone else. By contrast, looking at a child's abilities within a strength-based framework removes the sense of being out of control and out of options. Thus a teacher's mindset is often a very crucial influence on a student's adaptation, as children can be very perceptive in sensing the reactions of teachers and others who interact with them.

The power of mindsets was evident in a study conducted in the 1960s by social psychologist Robert Rosenthal. In that study, teachers were given lists of students who they were told had done well on academic testing and were likely to succeed in the classroom. At the end of the school year, the students who were on these lists did indeed do better academically than the students who were not on the lists. However, the lists the teachers were given included just randomized names of students. Although this experiment was subsequently criticized on methodological grounds, it raises the point that if children are expected to succeed (or, conversely, to fail), the adults who hold these expectations may well be relating to them (knowingly or unknowingly) in ways that reinforce the expectations, and thus creating a self-fulfilling prophecy (Rosenthal & Jacobson, 1992).

Clinical Case Example: Jeremy

I chaired another CSE meeting for a sixth-grade boy named Jeremy, who had been diagnosed with ADHD as well as several learning challenges. As the meeting started, I could immediately sense that both parents took a very negative view of their son. They spoke about his poor motivation for school, his tendency to lie and steal (he had been accused of stealing an exam at school, but it could never be proven), and their overall lack of trust in him. The teachers then joined in, going along with the parents' criticism of this youngster. It felt as if all the adults were looking for this opportunity to express their anger and frustration. As the meeting unfolded, I began to think about how a strength-based approach could be applied to this situation.

Admittedly, I felt outnumbered by the other participants in the meeting, as the tone was so negative you could feel the hostility in the air. I then decided to take the risk and asked the entire group what assets they felt this boy had. I prefaced this question by saying that I was going to ask something that was not consistent with what was being discussed, and I wanted everyone to consider it carefully before responding. Not one participant, including Jeremy's parents, could provide an answer. I then mentioned that his intelligence testing definitely showed areas of strength. This did not get any response. I then reflected how difficult it must be for Jeremy if the main adults in his life, parents and teachers, were saying they didn't trust him or see him as capable.

At this point the room fell silent. The parents then said that all Jeremy did in his free time was play video games and look on various websites for ways to win. The parents then went on to say that Jeremy had recently developed an interest in magic, but they felt that this interfered with his studies. I responded that these were two opportunities to capitalize on his strengths. I suggested to his parents that they make time each day to watch Jeremy perform magic as he taught himself tricks from the Internet. I also suggested that since he was so adept at finding ways to "beat" his video games, he should be encouraged to write his discoveries down in book form, and even to share this book with the class. This would not only help establish Jeremy's sense of competence and improve his interactions with others, but also develop his written language skills.

At this point, there was a marked change in the atmosphere. This seemed to free the other people in the room to begin to come up with ideas to promote Jeremy's strengths and competencies. In fact, one teacher offered to help Jeremy write a book and bind it. As it turned out, the group came up with a very long list of ideas, and the meeting ended with a very different tone than it began with.

As in the case of Dawn, this meeting was very powerful. As Jeremy's meeting began, it felt to me that a "piling-on" mentality was developing, as the parents and teachers had joined forces to highlight Jeremy's shortcomings and this dynamic was gaining momentum. I was thinking that the anger all parties were demonstrating toward Jeremy was probably reflective of how he experienced these primary adults in his life. In an effort to prevent this anger from continuing, I then asked the group what assets they believed Jeremy had; when no one could provide a response, I then reflected how difficult life must be for this young man. My goal in making this observation was to allow the participants to become more empathic and consider Jeremy's perspective.

As the meeting unfolded, it became apparent that my comments were having the desired effect. A gradual shift occurred as parents and teachers began to view Jeremy as a struggling and vulnerable child, as opposed to someone who was unmotivated and oppositional. In short, the entire group's mindset began to change. Just as in Dawn's case, this allowed Jeremy's teachers and parents to begin acknowledging Jeremy's strengths. When the parents first mentioned Jeremy's talents in performing magic and playing video games, it was likely that the participants did not initially view these as means to build up Jeremy's self-esteem and to alter the interactions they had with him. However, during the course of the meeting, these interests were presented as islands of competence. Although some readers may argue that the nature of what was discussed was beyond the scope of what school meetings should cover, I would strongly disagree. Positive psychology encourages creativity and "thinking outside the box" when designing interventions. The ultimate goal of the strategies offered was to help Jeremy take the first steps to experience success, both academically and behaviorally. It is interesting to note that the parents and teachers did follow through on the suggestions offered. Jeremy did write a handbook with the help of his teacher, and his parents worked on changing their interaction with him by shifting their focus to the things he did well. In fact, for the balance of the school year Jeremy's grades improved, as did his behavior both at home and at school. Nearly 2 years later, Jeremy continued to experience success as he became an honor roll student.

CONCLUDING COMMENTS

A major benefit of the strength-based model is that not only can children benefit from the strategies utilized, but adults have opportunities to reexamine their mindsets. This is very important, as children can be very perceptive in reading their teachers (and parents), and their behaviors will often unfold in response to how they experience the adults in their lives. I view this model as a collaboration among myself, students, staff members, and families, as it does not put the burden solely on students to change their behavior, but allows others to participate actively in the change process. Thus it is a model of empowerment for all. Working in this way allows all of the adults involved to serve as charismatic adults for children, as we work together to develop their islands of competence as well as enhance their self-esteem. For me, seeing children and adults become more optimistic and hopeful has been a very potent experience, which further reinforces my adherence to this model. The late humanitarian Nelson Mandela eloquently captured the essence of the strength-based model when he said, "The greatest glory in living lies not in never falling, but in rising every time we fall" (*www.goodreads.com/quotes/122796-the-greatest-glory-in-living-lies-not-in-never-falling*).

REFERENCES

19 minutes—how long working parents give their children. (2014). *Daily Mail.* Retrieved from *www.dailymail.co.uk/news/article-396609/19-minutes—long-working-parents-children.html.*

Avramidis, E., & Norwich, B. (2002). Teachers' attitudes towards integration/inclusion: A review of the literature. *European Journal of Special Needs Education, 17*(2), 129–149.

Brooks, R. (2003). Further thoughts about personal control. Retrieved from *www. drrobertbrooks.com/monthly_articles/0302*.

Brooks, R., & Goldstein, S. (2001). *Raising resilient children: Fostering strength, hope, And optimism in your child*. Chicago: Contemporary Books.

Brooks, R., & Goldstein, S. (2002). *Nurturing resilience in our children: Answers to the most important parenting questions*. Chicago: Contemporary Books.

Goodyear-Brown, P. (2012, March). *Creative play therapy interventions for problems of dysregulation*. Presentation at the thirteenth annual conference of the New York Association of Play Therapy, New York.

Crenshaw, D. A. (Ed.). (2010). *Reverence in healing: Honoring strengths without trivializing suffering*. Lanham, MD: Jason Aronson.

Goldstein, S., & Brooks, R. B. (2013). *Handbook of resilience in children* (2nd ed.). New York: Springer.

Hayes, B. (2013, July 25). Top ten problems facing public education in America [Blog post]. Retrieved from *www.gimby.org*.

Mann, D. (2013, December 4). More than 6 percent of U.S. teens take psychiatric meds: Survey. Retrieved from *www.consumer.healthday.com/kids-health-information-23/adolescents-and-teen-health-news-719*.

Masten, A. (2001). Ordinary magic: Resilience processes in development. *American Psychologist, 56*, 227–238.

Masten, A. S., Herbers, J. E., Cutuli, J. J., & Lafavor, T. L. (2008). Promoting competence and resilience in the school context. *Professional School Counseling, 12*, 76–84.

Ricks, D. (2013, May 13). CDC: 1 in 5 kids has mental health issue. *Newsday*. Retrieved from *www.newsday.com/news/health/cdc-1-in-5-kids-has-mental-health-disorder-1.5279380*.

Rosenthal, R., & Jacobson, L. (1992). *Pygmalion in the classroom: Teacher expectations and pupil's intellectual development* (rev. ed.). New York: Irvington.

Rumberger, R. (2013). Poverty and high school dropouts. Retrieved from *www. apa.org/pi/ses/resources/indicator/2013/05/poverty-dropouts.aspx*.

Stargell, W. (1983, April 3). Yes, I am ready. *Parade*, p. 10.

Swanbrow, D. (2004). U.S. children and teens spend more time on academics. Retrieved from *www.ur.umich.edu/0405/Dec06_04/20.shtml*.

U.S. Department of Education, National Center for Education Statistics. (2013). Indicators of school crime and safety: 2013. Indicator 17: Students' perceptions of personal safety at school and away from school. Retrieved from *www. nces.ed.gov/programs/crimeindicators/crimeindicators2013/ind_17.asp*.

Chapter 8

Enhancing Resilience through Play Therapy with Child and Family Survivors of Mass Trauma

RISË VANFLEET
CLAUDIO MOCHI

Traumatic events are part of life. They occur in all countries and throughout history. The nature of these events can be quite different: natural disasters such as hurricanes, tornadoes, fires, or earthquakes; or human-made disasters such as armed conflict and wars, community shootings, industrial accidents, genocide, or terrorism. Traumatic events can occur at more local levels as well, such as house fires, car accidents, or medical emergencies. Most people will experience traumatic events in their lives, and those who do not are very likely to be exposed to them through instantaneous reporting on television and other news media. "Mass trauma," in which whole communities or regions are affected by a disaster, is particularly challenging because the infrastructure is often destroyed, and people's access to resources is eliminated. This chapter is designed to provide an understanding of the needs of communities of people (especially children and parents) in such situations; a template for intervening soon after such an event; and the importance of play and play therapy for capitalizing on and building resilience in children and families, both immediately after a disaster and long into the future.

The use of center-based play therapy or family therapy comes later in the intervention process after disasters strike. In the days, weeks, and months following a disaster, families' needs are often more closely related to survival than to psychological welfare. Even so, some forms of play intervention can be employed "in the field" to ease the stress on children and their families, and to make connections that can lead to the implementation of more traditional play therapy services at a later time.

The type of play intervention or therapy needed depends greatly on the nature of the disaster; the pre- and postdisaster functioning of the family and community; the resources that are available; the skill levels of local helpers; the length of time that has passed since the traumatic event; and the types of assistance (if any) that have been provided since the event. Ongoing disasters, such as wars and refugee situations, require a different approach from events that have ended, such as tornadoes or hurricanes. Play therapists and mental health professionals often play different roles, depending on these circumstances and time frames. In addition, when practitioners arrive from outside the community, their roles can be quite different from those of practitioners who reside in the affected community.

This chapter briefly outlines the impact of disasters on the psychosocial well-being of survivors; describes appropriate roles for play therapists and other mental health professionals; highlights the importance of play in the disaster context; and provides examples of play-based interventions that can be conducted in the field soon after mass disasters, as well as more traditionally delivered play therapy interventions that can be applied to help children and their families later in the process of disaster recovery.

INDIVIDUALS FACING CRITICAL EVENTS

Traumatic events often generate intense fear, physical injury, and life-threatening circumstances. They are not exceptional in a statistical sense, with one study finding that 68% of children under the age of 16 had experienced some sort of traumatic event (Copeland, Keeler, Angold, & Costello, 2007). On the other hand, traumatic experiences challenge individuals' and communities' adaptive responses, imposing very difficult obstacles to coping and frequently upsetting their psychological, social, and emotional balance. Mochi (2009) has commented that "Every situation that exceeds one's capability to adapt produces anxiety which can interfere with the individual's normal functioning" (p. 71), but not all traumatic events have the same impact. As the lack of control and of predictability increases, so does the likelihood of greater impact on the people involved (McFarlane & De Girolamo, 1996). When people's usual coping methods are inadequate to a situation, they are likely to feel vulnerable and unprotected. Experiencing traumatic events, especially when there is a high level of exposure or lengthy duration of the event, leads to feelings of helplessness and hopelessness (Pynoos, Steinberg, & Goenjian, 1996). These feelings can persist for a very long time.

I (Claudio Mochi) was involved with the assessment of the psychosocial condition of Serbian citizens who had fled from their homes as a consequence of the 1990s Balkan conflicts (i.e., these Serbians were internally displaced people). The assessment (Mochi & Ljubomirovic, 2003) was motivated by the failure of prior programs that had focused on rental payments, microfinancing, and house-building programs. Data were collected for several months and in six different living centers for these displaced people. The results showed that the majority of the adults felt no hope for the future 7–12 years after the war. They reported day after day that there were no services planned or performed to improve their poor living conditions. They had reached a point where they believed that there was nothing they could do to improve their circumstances, and it was meaningless to try any longer. They had completely lost hope. This is consistent with reports in the literature (McFarlane & De Girolamo, 1996) that "chronic and unpredictable stress may be more likely to create a series of enduring personality changes and disrupt the individual's basic sense of trust in relationship and confidence in the future" (p. 138).

At the same time, other individuals who had suffered the same circumstances were actively involved in improving their living conditions; in some cases, these persons were more deeply involved in making improvements than were some of the aid workers sent there to help them. Other researchers have also noted these vastly different reactions to similar situations. McFarlane and Yehuda (1996) have written, "Exposure to extreme stress can produce personal growth and lead to increased self-respect" (p. 173). Others have observed the presence of "more confidence, enhanced relationships, deeper compassion and greater maturity" (Stewart, Echterling, & Mochi, 2014, p. 375).

This suggests that there is not an immediate or simple causal relationship between a disaster and chronic problems. Similar circumstances during a traumatic event do not lead necessarily to the same results because there are always variations in individuals' experiences, perceptions, coping abilities, and other factors (McFarlane & Yehuda, 1996; Ursano, Grieger, & McCarroll, 1996). Garbarino, Kostelny, and

Dubrow (1991) emphasize that objective and subjective danger are only weakly correlated. People coping with a disaster have their own unique sets of capacities, skills, experiences, and sensitivities, which can render them more or less vulnerable to the impact of the event. Some factors that play roles in coping and resilience include prior mental health issues, family history, predisaster stress levels, prior experience with similar situations, effectiveness of actions taken, degree of physical helplessness during the event, and events occurring in the aftermath of the disaster, among others (Eth & Pynoos, 1985; Frederick, 1985; McFarlane & De Girolamo, 1996; McFarlane & Yehuda, 1996; Pynoos et al., 1996).

In particular, the experiences that people have after a disaster can have a large impact on coping. Some people's psychological responses are triggered by continual reminders of what has happened and the losses they have endured. Others may live in isolated areas without access to food, hygienic facilities, or safe shelter. Still others struggle with the loss of their jobs, the inability to move freely, and/or the lack of opportunity to take action. When disaster situations last for long periods ranging from weeks to years, people must remain vigilant for new signs of danger, possibly increasing their posttrauma symptoms of hypervigilance when the trauma has finally ended. For those who are able to find physical safety and sufficient resources for survival (food, shelter, clothing, clean water, bedding), along with social support from other survivors or helpers, the possibility of fewer or less serious trauma symptoms becomes apparent.

CHILDREN FACING CRITICAL EVENTS

Just as adults do, children may show resilience during disasters, but they remain vulnerable to both short- and long-term trauma reactions. By virtue of having fewer life experiences, they usually have developed fewer coping mechanisms, so they are more heavily challenged to cope with traumatic events. Their reactions can be considerably influenced by those of their parents, teachers, and other adults around them as well (VanFleet & Sniscak, 2003). Children's posttrauma reactions show similarity to those of adults: agitation, anxiety, difficulty concentrating, anger or aggressiveness, nightmares, separation anxiety, being easily startled by noises or other triggers, regression, talking excessively or not at all about the event, changes in social relationships, and episodes of rage or numbness. Perhaps one of the most telling signs in children is the least well defined: Parents or teachers say that a child is "different" from before, or that something seems "off" (VanFleet & Sniscak, 2003). It is also important to remember that sometimes children begin to show symptoms of trauma reactions months after appearing initially to make a good postdisaster adjustment (VanFleet, 1998, 2011).

For children, too, there are many factors that influence postdisaster reactions: a child's age, developmental level, and cognitive ability to process complex information; the child's personality and other individual attributes; the nature, intensity, and duration of the trauma; the child's exposure to the trauma (i.e., how direct the child's experience of it was); the child's support network; the quality of the child's pretrauma relationships and general adjustment; and the presence and quantity of other stressors in the child's life (Garbarino et al., 1991; Hurrelmann & Lösel, 1990; Schaefer, 1994; Shelby, 2000; VanFleet & Sniscak, 2003). In general, children are more vulnerable to trauma than adults are. Since Lenore Terr's (1990) groundbreaking research about childhood trauma, much has been learned about the potentially serious and long-lasting impact of traumatic events on children's development and mental health (Garbarino et al., 1991; Garbarino, Dubrow, Kostelny, & Pardo, 1992; Gil, 2010; La Greca, Silverman, Vernberg, & Roberts, 2002; Perry & Szalavitz, 2010; Webb, 2007). Common child reactions to traumatic stress include feelings of helplessness/hopelessness, somatic complaints, poor emotional and behavioral regulation, distortions in perceptions of self and others, confused sense of identity, fearfulness, separation anxiety, aggression, guilt/shame, avoidance, night terrors, and attachment problems (Briere & Spinazzola, 2005; Garbarino et al., 1991, 1992; Gil, 2010; Perry & Szalavitz, 2010; van der Kolk, Roth, Pelcovitz, Sunday, & Spinazzola, 2005; Webb, 2007)

THE GOALS OF INTERVENTION
AFTER MASS TRAUMA

In any mass disaster, there is great variability in the ways that people respond, and those responses can vary over time as well (Mochi & VanFleet, 2009). This is true for both adults and children. In any disaster, there are risk factors that increase the chances of traumatization and poorer outcomes, and there are protective factors that insulate individuals from some of the bad effects. These are unique to each individual's situation. In many cases, the primary goal of intervention is to enhance the protective factors that are present and that can ameliorate individuals' traumatic responses (Ginsburg, 2011; Neenan, 2009; Reich, Zautra, & Hall, 2010).

The American Psychological Association (2014) has drawn 10 factors from the research that suggest ways to build resilience. Briefly, they include the following actions: (1) Maintain healthy, supportive relationships; (2) resist thinking of the crisis as "unbearable"; (3) accept those things that cannot be changed; (4) develop realistic goals, and break them down into steps for achieving them; (5) take action; (6) use the crisis to learn more about oneself and life; (7) develop self-confidence; (8) keep the broader context in mind, and develop a longer-term view; (9) maintain hopefulness—think about wishes for the future; and (10) take care of one's body and mind as best as possible—don't neglect one's own needs. Ginsburg (2011) has looked more specifically at the needs of children, calling the supportive strategies for building resilience "the seven crucial C's." He lists these as competence, confidence, connection, character, contribution, coping, and control. These concepts fit well within a postdisaster paradigm, and many of them are illustrated in the sections of this chapter outlining interventions.

Of the protective factors or support strategies that contribute to resilience, the most important component for coping with mass disaster involves relationships (Garbarino et al, 1991, 1992; VanFleet & Sniscak, 2003). Feeling connected with one's family or friends, or with other caring individuals on whom one can rely for support, is critical. McCubbin and Figley (1989) have suggested 11 factors associated with greater family resilience during and after trauma, based on their research. There is overlap with the factors listed in the previous paragraph, but each of these reflects how the family as a whole responds: (1) acceptance of the stressor without denial; (2) a family-centered response to the problem, rather than using blame or expecting one family member to "fix" things; (3) problem solving that focuses on finding solutions; (4) tolerance and patience with each other; (5) open communication about caring for each other; (6) high levels of communication with each other; (7) family cohesion; (8) flexibility in family roles and tasks; (9) efficient use of available resources; (10) absence of violence in the family; and (11) low levels of substance abuse or reliance on substances for stress reduction within the family.

Coping with the enormous challenges faced by children, adults, families, and communities during mass disasters is a complex and ongoing process. Much of the early work simply cannot be done in a mental health center or office. A community psychology approach provides a useful frame within which mental health and play therapy professionals can offer their knowledge, skills, and talents to aid the victims. The rest of this chapter focuses on processes and interventions that can be helpful, along with information about the timing of therapeutic interventions that are likely to benefit children and their families.

PREINTERVENTION CONSIDERATIONS

This section outlines the situations that mental health practitioners might face during the early stages after a disaster, as well as ways to think about and organize personnel and resources.

Professional Preparation

I (Claudio Mochi) kept in touch with a number of families with whom I had worked after a large earthquake in Italy. Seven years after the disaster, the families invited me back to the area for a special commemoration. As I walked through the temporary village in which they were located, I was struck by the number of people who remembered me, even when they had not been directly involved with me. The survivors of this community then shared something important: "Do you remember those psychologists [mentioning some of them by name]? They came here, applied their techniques at the school, scared our children even further, and then left, not to be seen again." Others said, "It took time to calm our children back down after they were here. I'm still angry and wish I could sue them. It was unfair for them to do that. Nobody was prepared for what they did, and they did not ask our permission to do it!" The intervention to which these survivors referred was probably conducted with good intentions, but somehow it had gone very wrong from the survivor community's point of view. These colleagues had received permission from a government school agency to provide the intervention, had conducted it in less than a week, and had then left. They had failed to take several factors into account: that the needs of children and the community at large are multidimensional; that there are different stages in the adaptation and recovery process following a highly stressful situation; that people's reactions are highly individual; and that after a disaster, most people will find a sense of security, release, and support mostly through trusting relationships.

It is not uncommon for mental health professionals outside a disaster region to want to help, and sometimes they "self-deploy," meaning that they do not wait for an invitation or coordinate their work with that of the emergency organizations overseeing the relief efforts. This is not useful. In other cases, they may be invited, but they deliver their services or interventions much as they might in a non-disaster-related environment or in their offices, without regard for what the survivors really need the most at the time. This is also not particularly helpful and in fact can be counterproductive. Finally, short-term bursts of intervention after which the professionals leave the area, not to be seen again, can be damaging. Survivors need continuity in their relationships with professionals; empathy and engagement; coordinated practical help; and interventions that recognize variation among and within individuals, as well as changes in needs over time.

Being a licensed professional or registered play therapist with a will to help is not enough. Guidelines drawn from the Inter-Agency Standing Committee (2007) designed to strengthen coordination of humanitarian assistance can be summarized as follows. A professional who is genuinely motivated to take part in any postdisaster intervention should follow certain requirements, such as (1) getting the proper training, (2) obtaining relevant experience, (3) being grounded locally, and (4) working within a structure that can ensure the intervention's duration and guide its perspective. It is important that any professional working in a posttrauma situation be an "added value." Everything that occurs after a disaster can either make the situation easier for survivors, or make things more complicated or worse. To be an "added value" resource, one must have appropriate training specific to disaster relief. Moreover, because isolated interventions can be seriously counterproductive, it is absolutely essential for professionals to work in coordination with local agencies and the survivor community. This also ensures that their interventions meet actual needs, are culturally attuned, and are effective and sustainable.

Professional Roles

With these key factors in mind, one must consider the roles that play therapists and other mental health professionals can play in disaster settings. If they are not from the local area and if they do not have the ability to assist on a regular basis over months or years, their roles are likely to be different. Even so, they can still serve as resources to the local community—perhaps by conducting training programs, providing consultations, or establishing programs run by helpers from the survivor community that can be operated into the future. As we have noted in an earlier publication,

> unless they are local, many post-disaster PT-Hs [play therapist-helpers] are on site for a limited period of time. Traditional play therapy is not possible or appropriate when therapists leave within a few weeks. No matter how well done, play interventions that end abruptly after a brief period run the risk of raising abandonment issues. (Mochi & VanFleet, 2009, p. 17)

Mochi and VanFleet (2009) go on to outline some of the roles that play therapists can assume in the postdisaster context when they do not have the capability of assisting for an extended period of time, such as conducting needs assessments, identifying helping resources within the survivor community, and training and consulting with local professionals and helpers as they conduct play interventions with children. Sometimes these roles are more important for the long-term than for the short-term well-being of children and families. The impact of disasters usually lasts for years, so play therapists who help create an ongoing system that continues to provide for the needs of children, parents, and the community are making a significant contribution. In many ways, postdisaster interventions should focus on creating a structured and enduring process. See Table 8.1 for a listing of possible postdisaster roles for mental health professionals, and questions one can use to determine the most suitable roles for particular professionals to play.

Assessment

Before significant play therapy or other mental health interventions can be implemented, it is important to assess needs from the survivor community's point of view. This process not only collects information that defines the most relevant interventions for that time period, but also engages people in the process and sets an inclusive, collaborative tone that establishes connection and initial support. Needs assessment meetings and informal conversations all supply important information and provide opportunities to offer empathic support. The processes of engaging survivors available to help with interventions, parents, and children are outlined in Mochi and VanFleet (2009), as well as in a document titled *Psychological First Aid: Field Operations Guide* (National Child Traumatic Stress Network & National Center for PTSD, 2007), and are not covered here due to space limitations. Just as initial assessment meetings are critical to the provision of high-quality play therapy for children and families in the office setting, so are these on-site assessment opportunities critical for the eventual implementation of any play therapy or family therapy program in the disaster context.

Early and ongoing assessments guide future intervention efforts. Assessments should not focus solely on psychological needs, as physical, medical, and survival needs are not only key in early days and weeks, but may affect people's ability to concentrate on their emotional well-being. Maslow's (1943) hierarchy of needs is a useful frame within which to conduct assessments. Assessments also need to be practical, with results that can be used right away. When I (Claudio Mochi) worked in Haiti

TABLE 8.1. Postdisaster Roles for Mental Health Professionals, and Questions for Determining Roles

Postdisaster roles	Questions for determining roles
• Coordinate with relief organizations	• "In a broad sense, what do you think you have to offer?"
• Provide physical and emotional support	• "What is needed most right now?"
• Assist with survival needs	• "What will be needed later?"
• Conduct needs assessments	• "Where can you do the most good?"
• Identify local helpers and resources	• "Will your work be 'added value'?"
• Help organize play-based group activities	• "How can you ensure that your work has sustainability?"
• Facilitate creative building or use of resources to meet needs	
• Train/supervise local helpers in professionals' areas of expertise, including play interventions	
• Conduct child, family, and community interventions	

for an extended period after the 2010 earthquake (as described below), I saw one large rescue organization use an evaluation tool that contained 187 questions. It took several months to complete, and the data were so extensive and complex that they could not be used at all. Finally, assessments should identify strengths and resources as much as they do deficits and problems. Each disaster has buried within it valuable resources that can be applied to assist with problems. Most play therapists have the capability and skills for using empathy in both formal meetings and informal conversations with members of the survivor community, to help establish trusting relationships, show caring and support, and gather information that can be used to ensure that interventions "fit" the community's needs at this time.

Early Support

The document *Psychological First Aid: Field Operations Guide* (National Child Traumatic Stress Network & National Center for PTSD, 2007) identifies core actions for mental health professionals to focus on during the early stages after a disaster. Among them are the need to establish human connections in a "nonintrusive, compassionate, and helpful manner," as well as to "enhance immediate and ongoing safety" while providing "physical and emotional comfort" (p. 19). This phase often requires at least several weeks after a mass disaster situation. This type of work bears little resemblance to traditional counseling or play therapy. The aid that is most valuable for survivors at this point requires the helping individuals to perform many different activities, all aimed at securing and stabilizing the situation, connecting with people, and assessing their ongoing needs.

When individuals feel unsafe, their abilities to function and process information are greatly reduced. Badenoch and Bogdan (2012) describe how the ability to connect with others is overridden by the need to focus on threat. It is critical, therefore, to create a sense of safety immediately. Similarly, a neuroscientist (Panksepp, 1998) suggests that when individuals feel unsafe, the flow of information and energy is related to fear, separation, panic, and rage. In contrast, Panksepp (1998) points out that when a sense of safety is established, it opens the possibility for people to connect with others by engaging several brain systems: the seeking system (curiosity, exploration, and enthusiasm/motivation); the care and bonding system (attachment and empathy); and the play system (the free-flowing, unstructured, uninhibited expression of joy).

There are many ways in which mental health professionals, including play therapists, can assist with creating safety, both physically and psychologically. They can help create interpersonal connections between survivors and themselves, but also within the community. Creating these connections allow interventions that point survivors in the direction of rebuilding and coping activities.

In 2005, I (Claudio Mochi) was involved in establishing a psychosocial center for children in Hebron, a city in the West Bank of Israel. Armed conflict was ongoing, and children were exposed to the sounds of detonations, helicopters flying overhead, and other reminders of the conflict close at hand. What seemed to reassure children the most was the calm, self-controlled behavior of my local colleague. Children looked to him to gauge their own safety. He was able to convey reassurance and support by modeling calm attitudes and behavioral skills. The power of relationship in establishing a sense of safety was pronounced in that situation (Mochi, 2009).

BUILDING RESILIENCE
IN THE EARLY DAYS AND WEEKS

Once a reasonable sense of safety and relationships with community members have been established, it is important for children—just as it is for adults—to have experiences that gradually increase their involvement, give them a sense of being capable and effective, and help them engage in their own and others' care. All of these factors coincide with the protective factors or elements of resilience covered earlier in this chapter. Some children are more readily engaged than others, but even withdrawn children should be involved by asking for their ideas, seeking their feedback about plans or activities, and providing them with news and updates.

"Play is an essential component of the recovery process. Play therapists recognize the power of play as a dynamic, life-affirming process that can be intrinsically fulfilling, thoroughly absorbing, and ultimately rewarding, especially in times of crisis" (Stewart et al., 2014, p. 371). For play therapists who are able to remain in the disaster region for a period of time, who can revisit it on a regular basis, or who are residents of the area themselves, it is a highly useful role to create and lead play-based activities for children, teens, and the community. These activities create the foundations of safety and relationships, as well as stress relief. They also provide further opportunities to assess how participants are coping.

In general, it is advisable to start with amusing, light-hearted activities that include local traditional play, games, or forms of entertainment, and that also bring together as many children as possible (as well as adults some of the time). The first activities should be relatively unstructured. It is very beneficial to engage the assistance of helpers and leaders from the survivor community in organizing events that involve just a few hours of play. The helpers, the leaders, and even the participants can be invited to plan the first program and to divide the various duties. For example, in the earthquake-stricken area of Leogane, Haiti, immediately after the assessment period, I (Claudio Mochi) and a number of Haitians eager to help organized two recreational activities per week. The local helpers agreed to prepare the space and the music. The aid organizations and the play therapist (myself) provided the toys and the refreshments. All those involved enjoyed dancing, playing, and laughing again. The full intervention in Haiti is described in more detail below.

As time goes by, and therapists and local helpers can see more clearly the needs that emerge during these less structured play events, they can begin to add more structured activities designed to enhance coping, build confidence, and strengthen problem solving and team building. Eventually, individual play therapy sessions may be possible, but these usually take place at a later stage. Training of local helpers and increased structure can be added as time goes by. Table 8.2 outlines the three levels of postdisaster intervention.

TABLE 8.2. Three Levels of Postdisaster Intervention

Level of intervention	Characteristics of intervention	Goals of intervention
Recreational activities	Traditional (for the culture), popular, light-hearted play, games, or sports as group activities. Planned and organized by the team or volunteers. Children can also organize activities under team supervision.	Fun, socialization, involvement in project activities, building relationship with team, identification of psychosocial needs, tension release.
Psychosocial activities	Age-specific group activities. Each addresses a specific goal. Each session is followed by a report to document the process/results.	Stress reduction, skills and abilities development, deeper needs assessment, coping strategies, problem solving, confidence development, greater sense of control, relationship building.
Play therapy	Individual, group, or family treatment using the therapeutic powers of play. For each individual/family, a treatment plan is established. Interventions may include nondirective, directive, group, and family play therapy modalities.	Addressing posttrauma reactions, other stress reactions, and problems not improved with psychosocial activities. Mastering trauma, building secure attachments, and enhancing healthy relationships.

Clinical Case Example: 2010 Earthquake in Haiti

Just a few months after the 2010 earthquake in Haiti, the assessment determined that a psychosocial program involving local and international organizations would be valuable. The project was designed as a community intervention, with the intention of including all residents of a village that was very close to the epicenter of the earthquake zone. The three levels of intervention pertaining to children included initial recreational activities (as described above), then progressive movement toward more specific and goal-oriented activities, culminating in individual play therapy sessions (VanFleet & Mochi, 2012). The local team was educated in all three levels of the intervention.

Two social workers, three psychologists, and several local helpers received training and began implementation of recreational activities, for which they received occasional supervision and training updates. Two hundred children participated enthusiastically in these activities, making it difficult to focus on various developmental needs of different age groups; supply sufficient water, snacks, and toys; and apply the concepts of child development and play-based treatment (many of which were quite new to these colleagues). As is necessary with most plans made in postdisaster work, adjustments were necessary. The plan to add more structured activities had to be delayed as the team attempted to "follow the lead" of the community of survivors, who seemed to be enjoying and benefiting from the less structured and more traditional Haitian forms of community music and play. The plan to conduct individual play therapy did not seem feasible at this time, and the program was clearly made more sustainable by focusing on the group activities. Goal areas for these play interventions were to reduce stress, increase community connection and engagement, provide coping skills, and build problem-solving abilities.

Clinical Case Example: 2004 Earthquake in Iran

After an earthquake that destroyed the city of Bam and several nearby villages in Iran, I (Claudio Mochi) was involved in developing several psychosocial centers where children and their parents could find some relief from the postdisaster stress.

In one of the villages, the first contact was made with a local leader (similar to a mayor) to inquire about her impression of needs, offer a program to people in her area, and ask her to suggest local people who might serve as helpers in the project. The plan was to involve adults with special skills and interests in children to support the team in managing the center. Decisions were gradually made about the location of the center; the area was cleared; and the helpers were then trained.

After an initial period of recreational activities, more focused initiatives began. Prior activities as well as parents' reports indicated that children were experiencing hyperarousal, with excessive vigilance, restlessness, aggressive behavior, irritability, and sleep disturbances. Plans were made for each group of children to participate in the program for at least 2 hours on alternate days. Boys ages 9–11 seemed to externalize their distress the most. Plans for this group focused on developing self-regulation, decreasing outbursts, and improving their relationships with each other (Mochi, 2004).

During the first hour of each 2-hour period, the local helpers provided calm activities involving both artistic and cognitive skills. The boys participated in drawing, painting, storytelling, and short reviews of academic subjects such as literature and math. During the second hour, the team, consisting of an Iranian psychologist and an Iranian social worker from elsewhere in Iran, provided focused play activities. This segment started with general, fun "icebreakers," followed by a more specific play-based intervention that focused on self-regulating and impulse control games, such as Red Light–Green Light, Musical Chairs, and Running Train. As the boys danced or ran around, they had to listen for various signals (whistles, music turning off, and others) that indicated that they were to change their activity or stand still.

The children enjoyed these activities and developed good relationships with the Iranian professionals who were running the interventions. The boys resisted leaving the sessions, however, and even resorted to throwing stones on one occasion when they were urged to leave. No one was injured, but this disruptive behavior was demoralizing for the team. It seemed that this level of intervention was insufficient to meet these boys' needs. Discussion of the problem included the mayor and other community representatives. This resulted in the addition of another local helper, a well-respected young man. An hour was added to each session, during which this young man planned athletic activities, with an emphasis on football (soccer). Beginning and ending rituals were established for this third hour. The beginning ritual involved doing physical exercises, and only those who listened to the instructions and took the exercises seriously were allowed to participate in the football game. This seemed to work well, and it appeared that the combination of play-based interventions followed by sports helped these children self-regulate much better. As this part of the plan evolved, the boys were provided with "official" jerseys, which reinforced the idea that they were part of a team and had a common goal.

This 3-hour program worked so well that it was then exported to the psychosocial centers in neighboring villages in the disaster zone, and a football tournament soon followed. This combined dynamic of play and physical opportunities for venting and expression within a well-contained structure helped modify children's behavior. They showed greater respect for the rules and dropped their aggressive interactions. All children experienced better relationships as a result. Children also cooperated more fully with planning more in-depth activities relating to their emotions and ways to recognize, express, and cope with these. No further distress reactions were reported by the parents or the community (Mochi, 2004).

BUILDING RESILIENCE IN THE MIDDLE STAGES

Although life after a mass disaster usually takes years to return to "normal," there are middle phases during which the initial shock passes and basic needs are mostly taken care of. Initial unstructured play interventions can now give way to more focused or goal-oriented play interventions. These can be conducted in groups of children, but those groups may be divided by age or goal area. Any number of group play therapy activities can be implemented at this time, as long as the needs of the children match the goals of the activity. Adventure-based activities and initiative problems can be particularly useful (Kottman, Ashby, & De Graaf, 2001; VanFleet, 2010).

Clinical Case Example: 2006 Earthquake in Pakistan

I (Claudio Mochi) was invited to serve as a consultant to support a process already begun in Pakistan several months after a major earthquake there. Psychosocial centers were in place, with the local community fairly involved. Some children were still experiencing symptoms of hypervigilance and unpredictable emotional reactions. An assessment showed the need for greater work on deeper emotions. Several play-based interventions, during which children drew and then talked about things that were resources for them and things that bothered them. This helped establish greater awareness of feelings, personal confidence, and mutual trust. After this, they were ready to take another step: facing challenges. The group participated in games that required them to use their problem-solving abilities and their initiative, but also to deal with frustrations that arose as they tried to solve the problems.

One example was a game called The Human Knot (Kottman et al., 2001). Each child in the group was asked to place one hand somewhere on a long rope. The children were then told that they needed to tie a knot in the middle of the rope without losing their grasp on the rope. After a few attempts, the children realized that the solution was not so easy, and they began to face frustration and feelings of failure. Tensions rose, and they had to face the difficulties with the task and each other. With persistence and some additional attempts, the children completed the task successfully. After the game, a short debriefing was held in which the children were guided to share how they felt during the activity, how they dealt with frustration and failure, what was useful in handling those difficulties, what contributed to their success, what might be helpful in similar situations, and what other coping mechanisms could be applied in frightening situations.

These types of goal-directed activities helped the children gain greater awareness of their feelings and how to express them, empowered them to solve some of their own problems, provided new coping skills, and added to their feelings of security and control. These children coped much better with subsequent aftershocks and other stressors in their lives. Nearly all of the children were supported during this period.

LATER STAGES IN THE PROCESS

As the postdisaster situation stabilizes and life begins to resume some semblance of normality, the nature of intervention often shifts as well. This shift may occur within several months of some disasters, and much longer afterward for others. Practitioners from other geographic areas who have worked in the disaster region far from their own homes are likely to have completed their roles in training the local professionals and helpers in how to continue working with children and families, or they may have seen the psychosocial help centers begin to function more independently. For these individuals, their role is likely to change to that of consultants. Those on-site helpers who are continuing the work may need case consultation or periodic, but less frequent meetings to guide their efforts. Nonresident play therapists remain available for support and occasional assistance, but their primary work is done.

For those practitioners who are working in their home communities, or who are able to continue their involvement on a regular basis, the focus may shift to ensuring the longevity of the programs and services they have created, and working with other clinicians and helpers to adjust to the needs of the children and families in the community at this time. A couple of examples follow.

Following the earthquake, tsunami, and nuclear disaster in the Tohoku region of Japan in 2011, Japanese psychologists and play therapists translated the Mochi and VanFleet (2009) article into Japanese and used it as a starting point to develop their own intervention plan for children of the region. They trained and supported teachers living in the affected areas in how to work effectively with children after a disaster, and how to employ play-based methods to help with trauma-related problems that arose and to prevent others from arising. This was done on a regular basis and has continued for the several years since the disaster (A. Ohnogi, personal communication, 2009–2013). They made visits to the teachers less frequently as the teachers became capable of handling the children's emotional needs more independently.

After the terrorist attacks of September 11, 2001, I (Risë VanFleet) was among several professionals invited to train and supervise play therapists, other mental health professionals, and educators in New York City and New Jersey in the use of play therapy, and particularly Filial Therapy (FT; VanFleet, 2014) for approximately a year. The training programs were conducted initially under the auspices of a local play therapy organization as well as the New York City Board of Education, and many of the early trainings were donated by the professionals involved. Later, as local professionals saw the value of these approaches, they independently requested further training and supervision. As their own competence and confidence grew, their need for subsequent training and supervision lessened. The use of FT after 9/11 is described in greater detail below.

After other disasters, the needs of the community change with time, and play therapists can assist with training of other key helpers or provide direct service if they are residents of the community. During Hurricane Katrina on the U.S. Gulf Coast in 2005, many families were displaced, and some settled in communities quite far away. As is often the case with such large-scale disasters, the process of rebuilding took years. I (Risë VanFleet) was invited approximately a year after the hurricane to one small city where many Katrina survivors had moved. There had been increasing tensions between the original residents and the displaced families, mostly because of child behavior problems in the schools and the community. Problems had begun surfacing with a number of the displaced children, and long-time residents were intimating that the "refugees" should go home. A consultation and brief training program for teachers helped put these problematic behaviors in the context of the disaster. This included the information that many children do not show symptoms until 6, 9, or even 12 months after a disaster. The teachers and some local mental health professionals were then able to see that many of the behavior problems these children were experiencing were probably posttrauma reactions, which helped shift their thinking about how the problems needed to be handled. They began to work on a school-based program in which the emotional needs of these children could be identified and assisted appropriately. The sense of relief among the workshop attendees was palpable.

Play Therapy in the Later Stages

During this later period after a mass disaster, child-centered play therapy (VanFleet, Sywulak, & Sniscak, 2010) can be very useful in establishing rapport and providing children with new opportunities to express their current concerns. By virtue of its nondirective nature, it is also helpful for identifying what issues might still be unresolved for a particular child. Specific directive and group play therapy techniques can be applied for specific goal areas. Numerous books about play therapy and play-based expressive techniques are now available (e.g., Drewes, Bratton, & Schaefer, 2011; Goodyear-Brown, 2005; Kaduson & Schaefer, 2001; Lowenstein, 1999). At this time, play therapy might well be offered at clinics, at schools, in hospitals, or even at psychosocial help centers that have been established earlier during the postdisaster period. Because basic survival needs have by now been more fully met, the forms of intervention begin to resemble the services that play therapists and other clinicians offer in their offices or communities. Again, it is important that clinicians working with children and families be from the disaster area so that continuity can be assured, while professionals assisting from other geographic areas can provide important training and supervision to help those doing the direct service work.

Filial Therapy in the Later Stages

FT, mentioned above (Guerney & Ryan, 2013; VanFleet, 2014), is a family therapy intervention that is very useful in the later stages of mass disasters. It can be provided to individual families experiencing residual trauma problems with their children, in groups that help families offer greater support to each other, and as a means of building resilience. It is not well suited to the early postdisaster stages because there are so many other needs that must be addressed at that time, and the middle stages often involve much rebuilding in both physical and psychological realms. But when the situation and the community have stabilized somewhat, FT provides a unique intervention that helps children play through their fears and trauma reactions in the context of their own families, while at the same time building upon (or rebuilding) the family cohesiveness and connections shown to be so critical for effective recovery from traumatic events (Figley, 1989; Garbarino et al., 1991, 1992; McCubbin & Figley, 1983; VanFleet & Sniscak, 2003). As the just-cited authors and researchers have noted, one of the most important features of disaster recovery and the establishment of resilience is the presence of strong, supportive family relationships. Also noted, however, is how difficult such strength and support can be for parents to provide when they themselves are deeply stressed by the disaster.

Often psychosocial help has been unavailable at earlier stages of the disaster, or it has been provided with some amelioration of the trauma's impact. Even so, strengthening families in such a way that they can continue to provide the secure attachments and opportunities for expression and resolution becomes much more feasible as the initial shock of the disaster begins to dissipate and families try to move on with their lives. As noted throughout this chapter, children often show trauma symptoms months after a disaster has occurred, and it is during this time period that FT is most feasible and beneficial to provide.

In FT, therapists train parents or other caregivers (including relatives, teachers, or helpers in the survival community) to provide one-to-one child-centered play sessions for their children. The parents learn to apply four primary skills: (1) "structuring," which is how a parent starts and ends the play sessions, conveying the concept that the child leads the way and the parent ensures a safe, contained environment; (2) "empathic listening," in which the parent briefly describes the child's play with a focus on the child's or the play characters' feelings, conveying acceptance of the child's play when the child is playing by him- or herself; (3) "child-centered imaginary play," in which the parent assumes and enacts pretend play roles that the child requests, often providing a unique attunement to the child's motivations, feelings, and wishes; and (4) "limit setting," in which parents apply a clear three-step approach (stating limits, giving a warning, and enforcing consequences if the child is not able to self-regulate). These skills work together to provide a unique environment that strengthens parent–child understanding and offers parents and children many opportunities for healing together.

After parents or caregivers are trained, they hold weekly half-hour sessions with each child in the family while under the direct supervision of a therapist. After parents have developed competence and confidence in conducting the play sessions with their children (typically after four to six supervised play sessions), they can continue them without direct supervision, but they still check in regularly with the therapist to ensure that the process is working as it should. Some FT groups continue long after the initial goals are met, and the members provide support to each other in a way that helps strengthen community ties.

An advantage to the use of FT in postdisaster situations is that it meets a variety of family needs through one family-focused intervention. Children work through their trauma reactions through the play sessions; parents understand their children's needs and feelings much better; and the parents feel empowered to help their children, and in so doing reduce their own feelings of helplessness. The parents support and help their children, while the therapist supports and helps the parents. FT has been clearly shown through 50 years of research to be effective in accomplishing these goals (VanFleet, 2014).

FT is valuable for building resilience in many ways. It builds parents' and children's sense of competence and confidence; it strengthens their connections within the family; it helps parents contribute to their children's healing; and it gives children and parents a greater sense of control (Ginsburg, 2011). Through this process, they develop coping strategies while working and playing together. The whole-family focus of FT directly addresses many of the resilience factors identified in the literature (Garbarino et al., 1991, 1992; McCubbin & Figley, 1983).

Clinical Case Example: Filial Therapy after 9/11

The clinicians trained fully in FT after the 9/11 attacks (see above) conducted FT at approximately the 6-month mark and after, with families affected by both the New York City and Pentagon acts of terrorism. Dozens of families took part, and I (Risë VanFleet) supervised many of the cases. Many parents reported how good it felt to be able to do something concrete to help their children, and they also indicated that the emotional and behavioral problems their children had experienced lessened considerably after they began their weekly play sessions. One mother noted, "At first I was worried about whether or not I could handle the traumatic play, but with my therapist's support, I was able to see how this process helped my children and me together. I felt stronger myself, knowing that I was helping my children cope with the unthinkable tragedy that happened to us." In one case, researchers studying the stress on families created by 9/11 asked a mother why she was able to be such a great model of healthy attachment during her experience of traumatic grief, and she simply said, "Filial Therapy." The researchers then asked her what that was, and she put them in touch with her therapist to learn more.

Therapists working with these families prepared the parents for potential trauma and mastery play during the training phase. In some cases, an extra mock play session was included to help the parents respond to scenes of falling buildings, plane crashes, and burial scenes. This was important not only to ensure their skillful responses to their children's play, but to help them discuss their own traumatic grief in anticipation of these play themes. Then, when such themes emerged, the parents knew how to handle them and could discuss them and their own feelings with the therapist afterward. For example, Timmy had lost his father in the World Trade Center. His early play sessions with his mother consisted of many plane crashes into buildings, followed by the deployment of toy fire trucks and ambulances. Although his mother found these scenes somewhat difficult to watch, her thorough preparation allowed her to provide empathic listening responses to this play without breaking down: "Another plane crash! And the building is going down! The people are very scared, but now the fire trucks are coming. They are trying to help the people." She was able to discuss her feelings afterward with the therapist; she commented that even though this play sometimes rekindled her own pain, the therapist's support helped her contain it during the play sessions, and she was very pleased to be able to help Timmy communicate about his fears. Later, Timmy asked his mother to help him bury people in the sand tray and arrange small displays of commemoration, using a variety of miniatures on top of the imaginary graves. His mother commented that she felt calm during this—that sharing this symbolic healing with her son made her feel better in many dimensions. FT helped strengthen the resilience of both mother and son through their deepening relationship.

Military families involved in multiple deployments immediately after 9/11 and in the years since then have also found FT to be very helpful. Some parents reported separation anxiety problems in their children and high levels of family stress during deployments, as well as during times when the service members returned home. The use of FT has helped their children feel more secure; has helped the parents in each family work together as a team, whether they are near each other or far apart; and has helped each family reintegrate as the parents have found ways to expand the play sessions into more playful interactions together, even when a service member is seriously injured. One father with traumatic head and body injuries learned to conduct the play sessions from his wheelchair. He told me (Risë VanFleet) that he had thought he was going to be worthless as a father, but that FT helped him see just how untrue that was:

"I was really, really down. I felt I had nothing left to give my kids. But when they lit up when we played together, even though I couldn't move around much at the time, it gave me hope."

Another father in a similar situation commented,

"It was touching to see my son play out the army themes, and themes of my getting hurt. What was most amazing to me was how tender he was in being the 'medic' who was going to fix me and the other soldiers in his play all up. In that moment, he actually *did* fix me up, at the same time I was able to help him come to grips with what had happened to me. I still get teared up when I think of that."

Clinical Case Example: Filial Therapy after Hurricane Katrina

Months after Hurricane Katrina, when many families remained displaced in New Orleans, a local therapist who had full training in FT returned to the city after her own displacement and helped trained a group of local therapists in FT. They all implemented FT while receiving regular supervision, and many found it very rewarding as they saw how eagerly the families participated and benefitted (VanFleet & McCann, 2007). Many of the FT play themes centered on imaginary hurricanes; moving from place to place; reenactments of rain and wind; and safety, rescue, and trauma mastery play. Again, parents reported how empowered they felt through being able to contribute to their own children's recovery while being supported by their therapists. The therapists were supported in turn by other FT professionals, who offered additional training and consultation as needed.

CONCLUDING COMMENTS

Mass disasters leave families, communities, and entire regions with a vast array of needs. Basic survival needs predominate in the early stages, but as the situation gradually becomes less chaotic, various play therapy and community interventions become both possible and beneficial. It is important to deliver these in a manner that ensures their continuity and longevity, so play therapists and other mental health professionals from outside the region affected by a disaster must often become teachers, serve as consultants, and play a number of other unconventional roles. Empowering the local community and the affected families becomes critical to counteract the helplessness that attends most disasters.

The specific types of interventions change over time and with the situation as well. It is critical that those helping in mass disaster situations understand not only counseling and play therapy strategies, but also postdisaster mental health care and the humanitarian organizations and processes that will be operating in the region for a long time after the disaster. This chapter has outlined some of the considerations for intervention in this complex environment, and has provided information about the different forms that play activities and therapies can take. It provides an overview of the process, while highlighting the great value of play interventions for promoting resilience in children and their families in a postdisaster situation.

REFERENCES

American Psychological Association. (2014). The road to resilience. Retrieved from *www.apa.org/helpcenter/road-resilience.aspx*

Badenoch, B., & Bogdan, N. (2012). Safety and connection. In L. Gallo-Lopez & L. C. Rubin (Eds.), *Play-based interventions for children and adolescents with autism spectrum disorders* (pp. 3–18). New York: Routledge.

Briere, J., & Spinazzola, J. (2005). Phenomenology and psychological assessment of complex posttraumatic states. *Journal of Traumatic Stress, 18*(5), 401–412.

Copeland, W. E., Keeler, G., Angold, A., & Costello, E. G. (2007). Traumatic events and posttaumatic stress in childhood. *Archives of General Psychiatry, 64*(5), 577–584.

Drewes, A., Bratton, S. C., & Schaefer, C. E. (Eds.). (2011). *Integrative play therapy.* Hoboken, NJ: Wiley.

Eth, S., & Pynoos, R. (Eds.). (1985). *Post-traumatic stress disorder in children.* Washington, DC: American Psychiatric Press.

Figley, C. R. (1989). *Helping traumatized families.* San Francisco: Jossey-Bass.

Frederick, C. J. (1985). Children traumatized by catastrophic situations. In S. Eth & R. S. Pynoos (Eds.), *Post-traumatic stress disorder in children* (pp. 73–99). Washington, DC: American Psychiatric Association.

Garbarino, J., Dubrow, N., Kostelny, K., & Pardo, C. (1992). *Children in danger: Coping with the consequences of community violence.* San Francisco: Jossey-Bass.

Garbarino, J., Kostelny, K., & Dubrow, N. (1991). What children can tell us about living in danger. *American Psychologist, 46*(4), 376–383.

Gil, E. (Ed.). (2010). *Working with children to heal interpersonal trauma: The power of play.* New York: Guilford Press.

Ginsburg, K. R. (2011). *Building resilience in children and teens: Giving kids roots and wings* (2nd ed.). Elk Grove Village, IL: American Academy of Pediatrics.

Goodyear-Brown, P. (2005). *Digging for buried treasure 2.* Nashville, TN: Paris and Me.

Guerney, L. F., & Ryan, V. M. (2013). *Group Filial Therapy: A complete guide to teaching parents to play therapeutically with their children.* London: Jessica Kingsley.

Hurrelmann, K., & Lösel, F. (Eds.). (1990). *Health hazards in adolescence.* Berlin: de Gruyter.

Inter-Agency Standing Committee. (2007). Guidelines on mental health and psychosocial support in emergency settings. Retrieved from *www.humanitarian-info.org/iasc.*

Kaduson, H. G., & Schaefer, C. E. (Eds.). (2001). *101 more favorite play therapy techniques.* Northvale, NJ: Jason Aronson.

Kottman, T., Ashby, J. A., & DeGraaf, D. (2001). *Adventures in guidance: How to integrate fun into your guidance program.* Alexandria, VA: American Counseling Association.

La Greca, A. M., Silverman, W. K., Vernberg, E. M., & Roberts, M. C. (Eds.). (2002). *Helping children cope with disasters and terrorism.* Washington, DC: American Psychological Association.

Lowenstein, L. (1999). *Creative interventions for troubled children and youth.* Toronto: Champion Press.

Maslow, A, (1943). A theory of human motivation. *Psychological Review, 50*(4). 370–396.

McCubbin, H. I., & Figley, C. R. (Eds.). (1983). *Stress and the family* (Vol. 1). New York: Brunner/Mazel.

McFarlane, A., & De Girolamo, G. (1996). The traumatic stressors and epidemiology of posttraumatic reactions. In B. A. van der Kolk, A. C. McFarlane, & L. Weisaeth (Eds.), *Traumatic stress: The effects of overwhelming experience on mind, body, and society* (pp. 129–154). New York: Guilford Press.

McFarlane, A., & Yehuda, R. (1996). Resilience, vulnerability and the course of posttraumatic reactions. In B. A. van der Kolk, A. C. McFarlane, & L. Weisaeth (Eds.), *Traumatic stress: The effects of overwhelming experience on mind, body, and society* (pp. 155–181). New York: Guilford Press.

Mochi, C. (2004). *Rapporto di fine missione.* Rome: Croce Rossa Italiana.

Mochi, C. (2009). Trauma repetition: Intervention in psychologically safe places. *Eastern Journal of Psychiatry, 12*, 73–80.

Mochi, C., & Ljubomirovic, N. (2003). *Assessment of IDPs and refugees living in a collective center in Pcnja District.* Brussels: Médicins sans Frontières.

Mochi, C., & VanFleet, R. (2009). Roles play therapists play: Post-disaster engagement and empowerment of survivors. *Play Therapy, 4*(4), 16–18.

National Child Traumatic Stress Network & National Center for PTSD. (2007). *Psychological first aid: Field operations guide* (2nd ed.). Rockville, MD: National Child Traumatic Stress Network. Retrieved from *www.nctsn.org/ sites/default/files/pfa/english/1-psyfirstaid_final_complete_manual.pdf.*

Neenan, M. (2009). *Developing resilience: A cognitive-behavioral approach.* New York: Routledge.

Panksepp, J. (1998). *Affective neuroscience: The foundations of human and animal emotion.* New York: Oxford University Press.

Pynoos, R. S., Steinberg, A. M., & Goenjian, A. (1996). Traumatic stress in childhood and adolescence: Recent developments and current controversies. In B. A. van der Kolk, A. C. McFarlane, & L. Weisaeth (Eds.), *Traumatic stress: The effects of overwhelming experience on mind, body, and society* (pp. 331–358). New York: Guilford Press.

Reich, J. W., Zautra, A. J., & Hall, J. S. (Eds.). (2010). *Handbook of adult resilience.* New York: Guilford Press.

Schaefer, C. E. (1994). Play therapy for psychic trauma in children. In K. J. O'Connor & C. E. Schaefer (Eds.), *Handbook of play therapy* (Vol. 2, pp. 297–318). New York: Wiley.

Shelby, J. S. (2000). Brief therapy with traumatized children: A developmental perspective. In H. G. Kaduson & C. E. Schaefer (Eds.), *Short-term play therapy for children* (pp. 69–104). New York, Guilford Press.

Stewart, A. L., Echterling, L., & Mochi, C. (2014). Disaster and crisis intervention: Roles play therapists play in promoting recovery. In D. A. Crenshaw & A. L. Stewart (Eds.), *Play therapy: A comprehensive guide to theory and practice* (pp. 370–384). New York: Guilford Press.

Szalavitz, M., & Perry, B. D. (2010). *Born for love: Why empathy is essential—and endangered.* New York: Morrow.

Terr, L. (1990). *Too scared to cry: How trauma affects children . . . and ultimately us all.* New York: Basic Books.

Ursano, R. J., Grieger, T. A., & McCarroll, J. E. (1996). Prevention of posttraumatic stress: Consultation, training and early treatment. In B. A. van der Kolk, A. C. McFarlane, & L. Weisaeth (Eds.), *Traumatic stress: The effects of overwhelming experience on mind, body, and society* (pp. 441–462). New York: Guilford Press.

van der Kolk, B. A., Roth, S., Pelcovitz, D., Sunday, S., & Spinazzola, J. (2005). Disorders of extreme stress: The empirical foundation for a complex adaptation to trauma. *Journal of Traumatic Stress, 18*(5), 389–399.

VanFleet, R. (1998). *Play therapy for traumatic events: Workshop manual.* Boiling Springs, PA: Play Therapy Press.

VanFleet, R. (2010). *Group play therapy manual.* Boiling Springs, PA: Play Therapy Press.

VanFleet, R. (2011). *Empowering children and families after traumatic events: Workshop manual.* Boiling Springs, PA: Play Therapy Press.

VanFleet, R. (2014). *Filial Therapy: Strengthening parent–child relationships through play* (3rd ed.). Sarasota, FL: Professional Resource Press.

VanFleet, R., & McCann, S. (2007). The road to recovery. *Play Therapy, 2*(3), 16–19.

VanFleet, R., & Mochi, C. (2012). *Post-trauma helplessness: Multidimensional play therapy roles for empowerment* [Training handout]. Boiling Springs, PA: Play Therapy Press.

VanFleet, R., & Sniscak, C. C. (2003). Filial Therapy for children exposed to traumatic events. In R. VanFleet & L. Guerney (Eds.), *Casebook of Filial Therapy* (pp. 113–137). Boiling Springs, PA: Play Therapy Press.

VanFleet, R., Sywulak, A. E., & Sniscak, C. C. (2010). *Child-centered play therapy.* New York: Guilford Press.

Webb, N. B. (Ed.). (2007). *Play therapy with children in crisis: Individual, group and family treatment* (3rd ed.). New York: Guilford Press.

Chapter 9

The Dance of Resilience and Attachment in High-Risk Mother–Infant Relationships

STEPHANIE CARNES
DAVID A. CRENSHAW

Positive caregiver–child (most often mother–child) interactions increase attachment security. Secure attachment in turn robustly contributes to resilience in the child. Secure attachment is the pattern most associated with resilience and other positive outcomes in both childhood and adulthood (Grossmann, Grossmann, & Kindler, 2005; Sroufe, 2005; Stewart, Whelan, & Pendleton, 2014). The ability of the parent or other caregiver to attune sensitively to the baby is especially critical in the first year of life (Siegel, 2012). Siegel (2012) has stated, "A parent's capacity to be sensitive to a child and provide contingent communication is based on her ability to perceive the child's signals, make sense of them, and respond in a timely and effective manner to them" (p. 318). If, for example, the baby cries because he/she is wet, contingent communication requires the parent to read the signal from the child accurately; to be able in this context to understand that the baby is wet, and not hungry or cold; and then to respond appropriately by changing the baby, while also soothing the baby's distress. This attunement of emotional states is the essence of nonverbal, contingent communication (Siegel, 2012) and lays important groundwork for resilience in the child.

Secure attachment does not provide absolute immunity from adversity in life. Stewart and colleagues (2014) recently opined, "While secure attachment patterns do not ensure good outcomes across the lifespan, or protect individuals from all forms and levels of stress, children with secure attachments tend to have more effective and satisfying relationships with parents, friends, and teachers than children with non-secure patterns do" (p. 37). In addition, they do better in social problem solving, are better able to repair relationship ruptures, are more successful in academic pursuits, have fewer academic problems, are less vulnerable to psychiatric problems, experience less trouble with the law, and become more successful parents themselves than nonsecure peers do (Grossmann et al., 2005; Sroufe, 2005; Stewart et al., 2014). Thus secure attachment in early life paves the way for resilience in future life, although the degree of resilience is determined by contextual factors and the circumstances of a person's life. There is enormous vulnerability in any human life, and even the best possible start in life does not fully fortify a person against extreme adversity.

Secure attachment patterns lead to adaptive and flexible neural connections and pathways, which form the neurobiological basis of resilience. Conversely, as Gaskill and Perry (2014) have explained, "When these important attachment patterns are compromised through multiple and chronic lapses within caregiving systems, crucial neural systems can be altered. This alteration negatively affects key competencies, such as the ability to regulate emotions and experiences" (p. 178). As many as 35% of children entering foster care exhibit attachment disorders, and as many as 38–40% of high-risk infant and toddler populations may have such disorders (Gaskill & Perry, 2014; Zeanah et al., 2004).

YOUNG MOTHERS WITH TRAUMA/ATTACHMENT HISTORIES

Children develop "social maps" (Garbarino & Crenshaw, 2008) based on their experience in the world. "Some children see themselves as powerful, secure countries surrounded by allies. Others see themselves as poor little islands, surrounded by an empty ocean or hostile enemies" (Garbarino & Crenshaw, 2008, p. 50). The first of these types of social maps is the result of early secure attachment experiences; it reflects the way securely attached infants understand the social environment. If an infant feels well cared for, safe, protected, and loved, the map is one of "basic trust"—which, as the psychoanalyst Erik Erikson (1959) explained, develops in the first 6 months of life. If the first 6 months of life are marked with inconsistent care or even worse, such as abuse and/or neglect, then the infant's social map will be one of "mistrust," in Erikson's terminology. Such an infant will view the world as unsafe, frightening, and unpredictable. Our human social maps continue to develop throughout life, based on our subsequent experiences in our social world and our relational experiences—but our relationships in the developmental years with primary attachment figures remain singularly important. In particular, if a teenage mother has missed out on the love, protection, safety, and security that lead to basic trust, and if her social map tells her that the world is a scary, dangerous place and that people are not to be trusted, how will she be able to raise a securely attached baby?

Daniel Siegel (2004, 2012; Siegel & Hartzell, 2003) has focused in depth on mothers with attachment histories of trauma and unresolved loss. One example of the kind of intrusion from past disappointments— or, in the extreme, trauma in attachment relationships—is the adult who has a "preoccupied" state of mind with respect to attachment (Siegel, 2012). This state of mind is a classification derived from the Adult Attachment Interview (Main, Goldwyn, & Hesse, 2003). Siegel (2012) has elaborated, "This preoccupied state is filled with emotional turmoil centering on attachment-related issues. Mental models of relationships will bias present perceptions and expectations, as we have seen, in such a way that these persons may create their own worst nightmare of uncertainty in their relationships with others, including their own children" (p. 130).

Even when children are privileged to enjoy secure relationships with primary attachment figures, exposure to violence in the community can alter their social maps. Siegel (2012) states, "The impact of violence on children may be complicated by the fact that their inherent mental models of the world as a safe place are directly affected by their witnessing of violence in the community" (p. 82). Relevant to the high-risk relationships of teen mothers with their babies is our own observation that many of the young mothers in our clinical work experienced disrupted early attachments and were also exposed to violence in the community. Many of these teen mothers have documented histories of physical abuse, sexual abuse, neglect, and/or exposure to domestic violence. The concepts of "complex trauma" (Cook et al., 2005; Courtois & Ford, 2009) and "developmental trauma disorder" (van der Kolk, 2005) most closely capture the wide range of symptoms and dysregulation stemming from cumulative histories replete with abuse, neglect, or other trauma. Developmental trauma occurs during childhood when the developmental process is unfolding; it entails exposure to multiple, cumulative traumatic events, typically of an interpersonal nature, and has an adverse impact on the course of development (Gregorowski & Seedat, 2013; van der Kolk, 2005).

As clinicians, we realize that the "trauma narrative" (Cohen, Mannarino, & Deblinger, 2006) for children who experience ongoing trauma or complex trauma is really a case of a "life narrative," rather than a story of discrete trauma events. Many teens in foster care, and especially those in residential placements, experience life as a continuous horror story—a nightmare that never ends. One essential part of that life narrative is the emotional story of removal from home (often multiple homes), which is often the beginning point for developing a conscious and explicit trauma narrative; creating such a narrative is considered an essential part of trauma-informed work. Research in neuroscience, attachment theory, and trauma-informed care indicates that creating a trauma narrative—being able to tell a cohesive story about what happened—is a pivotal step in the healing process (Malchiodi & Crenshaw, 2014).

THE "MOMMY AND ME" GROUP

In 2010, the Children's Home of Poughkeepsie (CHP) opened a Young Mothers Program for high-risk expectant teens and young women who were already parenting. The young women in the program frequently and vocally expressed a fierce desire to protect their children, as well as the sentiment that they did not wish to lose their babies to child protective services (CPS) or foster care. Despite this, the cottage staff frequently observed that the young mothers exhibited limited knowledge of appropriate parenting practices and, at times, a general ambivalence toward fulfilling the responsibilities and demands of parenthood. As a result of the attachment trauma that many of these young mothers had experienced early in their lives, bonding with their own children proved to be incredibly difficult. As we and the program staff observed the myriad risk factors associated with poor bonding and attachment in early childhood, the decision was made to form a "Mommy and Me" group. The group co-leaders (the two of us) hoped that this group, which began in the fall of 2012, would offer a relaxed, safe, and comfortable space where the mothers could share their experiences, offer support to one another, and (most importantly) engage in playful interactions with their babies to strengthen mother–child attachment.

Like most groups, the Mommy and Me group has progressed through several different phases of interaction and involvement. Since many of the young women in the Young Mothers Program had experienced turmoil and familial disruption as a result of CPS involvement, the initial phases of the group were characterized by substantial mistrust and suspicion about the group's purpose. Many voiced the opinion that the group was simply another opportunity to place them "under the microscope" of parenting scrutiny.

Suspicion and Apprehension

During this first phase of "suspicion and apprehension," which was observed for approximately the first 24 sessions, the young mothers attended the group consistently, but participated minimally. They preferred to sit on chairs or couches in the playroom and hold their babies, with some mothers placing their babies on the soft play mat. The mothers appeared tense and reluctant to interact with one another, us, or their babies. They seemed to prefer to observe us as we interacted with the babies, instead of playing with their own babies. They were generally reticent during group discussions on parenting issues, and even the more outspoken mothers in the group seemed almost afraid to speak.

Tentative Exploration

In the second phase, "tentative exploration," which was dominant from approximately the 25th to the 36th session, some of the mothers gradually began to engage in group activities. It was clear to us that this was uncharted territory for the mothers. Although many of them made the move to join their babies on the floor, and some even began to participate in the group discussions, they still seemed to prefer watching their babies to interacting with them. This is certainly understandable, as these young mothers had enjoyed few if any playful interactions with their own caregivers in their early lives. To address this, we interacted with the babies in a playful manner, to model this type of interaction for the young mothers. The mothers' anxiety and uncertainty were palpable during this stage of group interactions. The babies seemed to absorb this nervous energy and were frequently fussy and in need of soothing. Although in a tentative and halting way, some of the young mothers began engaging their babies (and sometimes even other babies) in playful interactions, laying the groundwork for greater security in attachments and thus enhancing resilience (Stewart et al., 2014).

Active Engagement

The third phase of the Mommy and Me group, "active engagement," began to appear after the 36th session, but in some mothers not until after 50 sessions. In this phase, the mothers began to engage more actively with their babies, their peers, and us as the group leaders. As they became comfortable with one another and with us, they began to bond with each other and share some of their concerns as young mothers in foster care. The young moms also started to interact playfully with their children, embracing some of the modeled techniques and approaches we had demonstrated in earlier phases of group work. Although most of the mothers now seemed to feel comfortable enough to engage with their babies in some way, the level of playful interaction varied substantially throughout the group.

As the group began to coalesce, the group discussions became richer and more animated. The young moms voiced concerns about issues related to their status as teen parents, including their fears of monitoring and criticism by CPS and of losing their babies as a result of parenting mistakes, as well as their wishes to protect their children from intimate-partner violence. The issue of domestic violence was especially pertinent to the majority of the group, and many voiced strong opinions about the significance of, and ways to cope with, violence in relationships. It should be noted that while the young mothers were fiercely protective of their own children and often voiced the desire to shield their children from any type of hardship, they did not show the same concern for their own safety and well-being. As is common in the cycle of domestic violence, they appeared to lack a self-protective instinct. However, their similar experiences in violent relationships seemed to serve as a medium for engaging and connecting with each other and with us in a safe, low-pressure, and nonjudgmental way.

Early in this phase, a group narrative based on shared experiences began to emerge. This increase in relational capacity in the young mothers fostered resilience because they began learning to draw on the social supports available to them (Jordan, 2013). Although the therapeutic power of this narrative was limited by the minimization, denial, and dismissiveness of some mothers, it was a significant positive development that a substantive level of group discussion emerged at all, given the significant mistrust that characterized the early stages of group work.

As explained by renowned psychoanalyst Walter Bonime (1989), any active declaration of trust from those whose sense of trust has been significantly damaged should be viewed as a monumental clinical breakthrough and a critical step in the process of healing and growth. As a result of the enhanced sense of trust that we had developed with the young mothers by this third phase of group work, we were able to incorporate aspects of psychoeducation into the group's agenda, including discussions on how attachment and bonding occur and why such attachment is so critical to early childhood development. We demonstrated playful interactions with the babies in the first stage, and encouraged and supported the young mothers throughout as they learned to interact with the babies on their own. The foundation of trust created in the first two phases enabled us to facilitate the increased disclosure and sharing in the third phase.

Since the main goal of the Mommy and Me group was (and still is) to promote and strengthen positive mother–child attachment, one distinct feature of the group has been the inclusion of a Facility Dog, with the permission of the young mothers. The dogs involved with the Mommy and Me group were first Ivy, and now Ace, who are both Golden Retrievers and service-trained dogs. As the title indicates, a Facility Dog is assigned to a facility instead of being assigned to work with a combat veteran or disabled individual, and each dog has received over 2 years of specialized training. The dogs are incredibly calm and knowledgeable, with over 80 commands in their "vocabulary." Unlike traditional therapy dogs, the CHP Facility Dogs have been trained and tested specifically to work safely with emotionally volatile teens and children as well as infants.

The Facility Dog program began in 2010 when the CHP required such a dog with specialized training to accompany three girls ages 5–15 as they testified in court against their alleged abusers. Rosie, a Golden Retriever who passed away in 2012, became the first dog in the history of the New York State legal system to be approved by a judge to accompany a young sexual abuse victim as she testified against her abuser. As a result of the incredibly powerful and positive effect that Rosie had on this child in a potentially traumatizing situation, the CHP now uses only service-trained dogs, both in the courtroom and in the therapy room. These dogs have played a pivotal role in the process of helping children and teens with complex trauma create trauma narratives for themselves (Crenshaw, 2011, 2012, 2014).

INDIVIDUAL TRAUMA-FOCUSED THERAPY

In developing the Young Mothers Program, we realized that the Mommy and Me group work focused on attachment and bonding between the teens and their babies would not be sufficient. Given the unresolved attachment status of the young mothers, trauma-focused individual therapy was deemed essential. In their research, Webster and Hackett (2007) found:

> Unresolved state of mind placed adolescents with a history of maltreatment at greater risk for the development of a number

of behavioral and emotional problems that have, at their core, impairments in self-regulation, impulse control and stress coping. This finding points to the importance of the adolescent[s'] resolving in a coherent and integrated fashion, their earlier traumas and losses. (p. 374)

Such resolution becomes critical when the adolescents are mothers, so as not to place their infants at risk of disorganized attachment (the children's version of unresolved attachment). Adolescents with unresolved loss and trauma are prone to frequent crises and tend not to connect their current feelings, thoughts, and behaviors to past losses and traumas (Bailey, Moran, & Pederson, 2007; Bernier & Dozier, 2002; Cook et al., 2005; van der Kolk, 2005; Webster & Hackett, 2007).

Features of the cognitive-behavioral approach can be helpful at certain stages of the therapeutic work with adolescent mothers with insecure states of mind, in developing the mothers' capacity for reflection and addressing the cognitive distortions and incoherencies of their narratives. The capacity for reflection and problem solving emphasized in cognitive approaches fosters resilience (Shure & Aberson, 2013). In our experience, however, a great deal of repair in the affective domain must precede the cognitive approaches. Allen Schore (2012), a pioneer in integrating social, biological, psychological, and psychoanalytic theory, has elucidated the key tenets of what he calls "modern attachment theory"; his work challenges the primacy of cognitive approaches over affective work in therapy theory and practice for the past two decades. Schore believes that the pendulum is beginning to swing back toward more attention to the emotional realm of experience. Support for this increasing emphasis on the affective domain comes from neuroscience research, particularly research on the Neurosequential Model of Therapeutics (NMT; Gaskill & Perry, 2014). As discussed by Crenshaw and Kelly (Chapter 4, this volume), the NMT is a guide to sequencing therapy, based on theory about levels of brain development. The model emphasizes the need to select therapeutic interventions in keeping with the lowest level of the brain that is dysregulated. Another important principle is that treatment must access the brain at the level at which trauma occurred. Interventions must activate this brain region. If, for example, trauma occurred very early in life, and the lower brain (brainstem, diencephalon) is dysregulated, it is unlikely that more language-/cognitive-based therapies are going to be effective.

At the present time, there is an absence of evidence-based treatments for complex trauma in children and adolescents. Our work has consisted of using the latest findings in interpersonal neurobiology to guide our therapy, with emphasis on nonverbal, sensory-based therapies to soothe and calm the brainstem and to make therapy safe. We view the therapeutic relationship and the supportive environment as offering the potential for developing attachment security in these young mothers, which in turn will enable them to promote greater attachment security in their babies. Part of this emotionally corrective experience stems from the safe haven provided by the therapeutic relationship, which provides the acceptance, warmth, and empathy that have been sorely lacking in the lives of these adolescent mothers. The acceptance, warmth, and empathy experienced in the therapeutic relationship in turn increase the young mothers' potential for showing greater acceptance, warmth, and empathy toward their babies. A significant degree of this emotionally corrective experience is mediated by nonverbal means. Greater attention has recently been given to the components of the therapeutic relationship that promote change, including sensitive attunement, warmth, and therapeutic presence (Crenshaw & Kenney-Noziska, 2014). The later stages of therapy, after the calming of the brainstem and the affective reparative experiences, allow for cognitive work; this work consists of modifying mistaken beliefs/assumptions and correcting distortions.

SUPPORT WITHIN THE SOCIAL ENVIRONMENT

We also knew from the inception of the Young Mothers Program that formal therapy (whether individual or group) alone would not be sufficient to address all the trauma issues. Webster and Hackett (2007) have stated:

> Given that an Unresolved state of mind is conceptualized as an attachment relationship disturbance, it is through supportive relationships that trauma and loss can be resolved. Ideally, resolution would be best accomplished by a concerted and coordinated effort from supportive caregivers, teachers, child welfare workers and mental health professionals. (p. 374)

Our program emphasizes a relationally rich environment, with caring and supportive adults available to the teen mothers around the clock to offer empathic and sensitive attunement to their needs, and to give them opportunities for breaks from the caregiving of their babies when they are frustrated or overwhelmed. All staff members in the program are trained extensively in a trauma-informed treatment approach called the Sanctuary Model (Bloom, 2000). The Sanctuary Model is a systems-level intervention that is based on principles of attachment and the latest concepts of and approaches to trauma. The entire organization is examined from top to bottom, to determine whether and how we can be more trauma-sensitive. Our entire staff (including the support and maintenance staff) is trained in the Sanctuary Model, to ensure that everyone on the CHP campus working with traumatized children shares basic knowledge about trauma, as well as a framework and language for understanding and communicating in helpful ways with and about these children. The training begins with an intensive 3-day focus on trauma and its impact on children, and is followed up regularly with additional trauma-informed training. The rich relational environment helps the young mothers expand their social skills, as well as their verbal skills; the increases in both skill sets contribute to enhanced resilience (Luthar & Zelazo, 2003; Prince-Embury, 2013).

CLINICAL CASE EXAMPLE: JAMIE

Jamie was a 15-year-old Hispanic mother from an urban area in the Northeast. She came to CHP as a result of her "incorrigible behaviors" (a direct quote from her placement order), which included shoplifting, running amok in the streets, and fighting. These behaviors, however, were directly linked to her family background and her own history of disrupted attachment. Jamie was born to a 15-year-old mother who wanted the status that came with being a gang member's "baby momma" more than she actually wanted to be a parent. When Jamie was a young child, her mother "needed a break" from her and sent her to reside with a great-aunt in a Southwestern state. When Jamie was 11, the great-aunt passed away, and she was returned to the Northeast. For the next several years, Jamie bounced between her mother and her grandmother, neither of whom was able to provide her with consistent nurturing, structure, and support. Her mother refused to assume legal custody of Jamie, and a lengthy court battle ensued.

Jamie came into the Young Mothers Program in the summer of 2013 when she was several months pregnant. She engaged quickly in therapy sessions, and seemed to relish the opportunity to be listened to and heard. She spoke about her tumultuous relationship with the baby's father, a gang member and drug user. She spoke minimally about her mother, who was listed in intake materials as her discharge resource, despite her limited involvement in Jamie's life. In the intake session, Jamie stated very simply, "My mother didn't raise me. She didn't do anything for me." She was frank about her mother's inconsistent involvement in her life; she attributed this to her mother's incredibly young age when she was born and her seemingly wavering desire to be a mother. To make matters worse, Jamie's mother had had three more children while Jamie was in the Southwest. While her mother was certainly not warm, nurturing, or even particularly kind to her three younger children, she met their needs and seemed to prioritize them. This exacerbated Jamie's sense of being repeatedly rejected by her mother throughout her life. As Jamie approached her baby's due date, her mother became more involved in her life, but not in the way that Jamie so desperately needed her to be. Although she would not call Jamie or visit her, she attended all of Jamie's prenatal appointments and often asked questions about the baby, quickly posting excited updates on Facebook pages about her grandchild-to-be. Jamie felt more and more as if her mother saw her as a vessel for delivering a grandchild, instead of as a valuable, lovable person in her own right. Jamie herself was excited about the birth of her child, but her expectations about parenthood seemed somewhat unrealistic. She struggled to understand the developmental stages of early childhood, and she seemed to become frustrated when she learned about the myriad responsibilities of a new parent. Moreover, the social worker and child care workers were concerned about her ability to bond with her baby, given her own disrupted, inconsistent attachment.

Jamie in the Mommy and Me Group

In early 2014, Jamie gave birth several months prematurely to a healthy but tiny baby boy named James. She began attending the Mommy and Me group almost immediately after her baby returned home from the hospital. Whereas many group members need weekly cajoling to attend the group, Jamie was eager to attend and even asked if she could begin attending before her baby was born. Despite her enthusiasm, her initial level of participation mirrored that of other group members. During the first months of her attendance, she used the group to size up new residents, show off James's new clothes, or make loud, boisterous jokes or comments to the peers from her cottage. About 2 months into her attendance, Jamie got involved in a fight with a peer after the peer "insulted" the sneakers that baby James was wearing.* Her group attendance appeared to be predominantly focused on keeping tabs on her peers and maintaining her unofficial title as the group "goofball."

---

*Through the Mommy and Me group, we began to learn that the babies' clothing—in particular, their footwear—carries enormous significance. When the babies wear the latest "Jordans" (Nike sneakers), the mothers explain, their peers know that they have money and that they "take good care" of their children. This initially baffled us, but to these moms, who have mostly grown up in poverty, allowing their children to wear passé clothing or shoes is synonymous with poor care and even neglect.

During these sessions, baby James would sit in his car seat or lie in her arms. She rarely if ever cuddled, kissed, or even spoke to him. Occasionally she would place him on the soft blanket on the play mat, but since she would remain sitting in the chair, he would become disoriented and alarmed and begin to wail. She would need to be encouraged to attend to him and soothe him. This could be viewed as part of the "suspicion and apprehension" stage of the group process. By essentially refusing to engage with James, Jamie avoided any sort of potential criticism from her peers or from us (the group leaders) for her uncertain mothering.

The cottage staff members who worked with Jamie frequently reported to us that Jamie preferred to pass her baby to the staff when he was being difficult instead of mothering him herself. They also expressed concern regarding her low frustration tolerance with James, which compounded our observations of her apparent lack of knowledge about how to interact lovingly with a newborn. During the next phase of group work, we attempted to model for Jamie ways in which she could spend "quality time" with her child, such as singing to him, cuddling him, or using rattles or other age-appropriate toys while on the soft play blanket. She began to slowly relinquish her role as group cut-up and began to appear more interested in learning about parenting. She also began to engage more with her peers in a positive way—asking questions about their babies and bonding over shared experiences, such as getting no sleep, losing pregnancy weight, or struggling to find the best formula.

Jamie's Trauma-Focused Individual Therapy

While Jamie's engagement in the Mommy and Me group was certainly an important contributor to her maturation and development as a positive parent, it should be viewed and analyzed in tandem with the therapeutic work that took place in weekly individual trauma-focused therapy sessions. Initially, Jamie used her individual sessions to complain about being in placement. Despite her inconsistent, challenging relationship with her mother, she frequently stated that her mother would soon be going through the process of obtaining guardianship of her, and that she would leave care to live with her afterward. As her individual therapist, I (Stephanie Carnes) joined with Jamie and suggested that it must feel awfully frustrating to have so little control over her life, especially when it meant leaving decision-making power to people who didn't know her well, such as social services workers or even her mother. I took a neutral stance toward Jamie's mother's involvement (or lack thereof) in her life, and asked Jamie to teach me what it had been like to grow up "in your shoes."

Jamie was responsive to this approach, and she and I began to explore her relationships with her mother and grandmother, both in their current forms and in the past. The common theme of Jamie's experience with her mother was a pervasive sense of being inherently and deeply unlovable. As many children in foster care do (especially those who have been bounced from caregiver to caregiver), Jamie seemed to view her mother's lack of nurturance and love as proof of her own unworthiness of love, instead of her mother's inability to convey love. Jamie also spoke about her experiences of being shuffled to different family members, but craving only her mother, or *a* mother who would love and accept her.

Not only did Jamie never get to experience the positive attachment that serves as a foundation for all successive relationships, but she also lacked the internalized concept of "home," or a place of safety, love, and acceptance (Crenshaw, 2013). In the few disastrous family sessions I attempted with Jamie and her mother, Ms. B repeatedly criticized Jamie for her parenting, her selection of clothing, her hairstyle, and even her postpartum weight. She was eager to lambast Jamie for her "incorrigible" behavior and quick to reiterate her expectation that should Jamie and her baby ever come to live with her, Jamie would be responsible for all cleaning, cooking, and care of her siblings. When I gently attempted to suggest more realistic expectations for a parenting teenager, Ms. B would whip out her cell phone and begin taking photos of herself or her grandson. When her younger children ran amok during the session, she would dispatch Jamie to corral them. Despite Jamie's numerous attempts to engage with her mother or even display affection toward her, Ms. B remained aloof, unsympathetic, and uninterested.

These short-lived attempts at family work provided critical material to examine in individual therapy sessions. Jamie frequently asked for impromptu therapy sessions immediately following sessions or visits with her mother (which typically occurred when Ms. B needed to sign consent forms or other documents at the agency), and these sessions were used to process her feelings about the visits and the ways in which she was affected by her mother's general indifference toward parenting. The main theme of these sessions was exploring Jamie's internalized sense of blame and culpability for her mother's indifference toward her. She and I used her relationship with her grandmother, with whom she enjoyed a positive, supportive bond, to challenge Jamie's sense of "assumed unlovability," since her grandmother clearly found her lovable, respectable, and worthy of nurturance.

Gradually Jamie began to express anger, disappointment, and frustration regarding her mother's inability to be a genuine parent. Often these appraisals of her painful interactions with her mother were followed by a simple statement: "James won't have to deal with this." Although, like most first-time moms, Jamie often needed support or instruction to meet James's needs, she was fiercely protective of him. By examining and understanding how her mother's parenting had affected her, Jamie not only became able to relinquish much of the sense of shame and guilt she carried with her; she also began to define the role she wished to have in her son's life. Although becoming pregnant at such a young age had not been part of her plan, Jamie learned that she could make purposeful, deliberate decisions early in James's life that would positively shape his experiences with her, and with the world around him for years to come. This feeling of being able to make purposeful, deliberate decisions is a major characteristic of resilient people (Shure, & Aberson, 2013). She and I spoke about what would have signaled to her that her mother loved her, and the ways in which James would *know* that she loved him.

Though Jamie initially pointed to material gifts as the best way to show love, such as the $50 bill her grandmother slipped into her birthday card or the $100 sneakers with which she outfitted James, she later suggested that perhaps monetary gestures were just substitutes for consistent, unwavering, unconditional love. Concepts of "parenting from the inside out" were subsequently incorporated into therapy sessions, as was the relationship between early attachment and subsequent childhood outcomes. For her son's sake, Jamie was determined to break the cycle of poor attachment, inconsistent nurturance, and general stress that had permeated her own relationship with her mother, and her mother's relationship with her grandmother.

Jamie was the only young mom to attend the most recent (at the time of writing) Mommy and Me group, since many of her peers had gone home for the Easter holiday. We gave her the opportunity to "take a rain check," since the group consisted of the two of us, Ace (the Facility Dog), James, and Jamie. Surprisingly, Jamie asked to stay, and even stayed longer than we expected. She seemed to relish the opportunity to speak about her experience as a young parent, and she was actively engaged with James. She took great delight in showing us a video she had recorded on her phone in which she made silly sounds, which caused James to giggle and shriek happily. She seemed proud when we explained that this was the sort of positive, playful interaction that would serve as a basis for James's attachment and development. This enhanced sense of confidence and capability is critical in the young mothers' journey to becoming attuned, positively attached caregivers, and also to attaining a sense of self-efficacy, which is inextricably linked to resilience (Goldstein & Brooks, 2013).

As illustrated in Jamie's case, the therapeutic work in individual sessions and the Mommy and Me group captured a critical moment in her healing process. In addition to the painful stigma of being "foster care kids," the teen moms in the Young Mothers Program shoulder a host of burdens specific to the attachment trauma that the great majority of them—like Jamie—have endured. They are incredibly angry, almost on a cellular level, and rightly so. As a result of their anger, they engage in acting-out (or, as described in Jamie's case, "incorrigible") behaviors. These behaviors serve as a distraction from and an outlet for this stored-up anger, and may also be used as a sort of protective barrier to keep away perceived threats to their safety and survival. In this way, acting out becomes a learned defensive mechanism born of attachment trauma and justified by successive negative experiences in the interpersonal context.

Despite their attempts to shut out those around them, these youngsters are far from immune to the perceptions others hold of them. On the contrary, they have internalized other people's negative reactions to them. For youth with attachment trauma, such negative perceptions are tantamount to being rejected once again, reinforcing the cycle of poor self-esteem, shame, guilt, and worthlessness associated with abuse, neglect, or abandonment. For these young moms, the expectations of parenthood are added to this already precarious sense of self and deep-seated wariness of interpersonal relationships. Without extensive therapeutic work to repair ruptured attachment, expecting a troubled young mother to attune to and meet the needs of her child—when her own needs have never been met by a caregiver—is unrealistic and even unfair.

CLINICAL CASE EXAMPLE: SHAMIRA

Shamira was a 20-year-old African American female who had come into foster care at the CHP at age 13, after being the family "whistle-blower" on her father's almost ritualistic physical, sexual, and emotional abuse of her and her six siblings, as well as physical abuse of her mother. As a result of her courageous decision to expose what was going on in her home, Shamira was rejected by both her mother, who sided with her father, and her extended family, who disagreed with her decision to speak up. Worse still, her father threatened her safety, and an order of protection was obtained against him. Shamira frequently stated in therapy sessions that she regretted having told the CPS worker about what was going on in her family because of the way that it changed her family's perceptions of her. Moreover, immediately before she arrived at the CHP, Shamira was the victim of a violent crime in her neighborhood. Upon arrival at the CHP, Shamira was diagnosed with both major depressive disorder and posttraumatic stress disorder, and her vastly diminished self-esteem was apparent. Throughout her time in foster care, Shamira was involved with a man 7 years her senior. When asked why this relationship had endured, she reported that this man, David, knew everything that she had been through and was still with her. At age 17, she became pregnant with his child. According to Shamira, the pregnancy was planned. As she simply explained it, "I wanted to have a family again."

At this time, Shamira moved from a residential program on campus to the Young Mothers Program. Shortly thereafter, she gave birth to a healthy baby girl named Sonia. After Sonia was born, Shamira began exhibiting serious mental health concerns, especially in her interactions with her baby. Although she had formed a positive, albeit tentative, therapeutic relationship with me (Stephanie Carnes) prior to Sonia's birth, therapy sessions after Sonia was born consisted of Shamira's staring blankly at me while remaining nonverbal. She seemed disconnected in the cottage as well. Child care staff frequently reported that Shamira would allow baby Sonia to cry for half an hour at a time while refusing to tend to her, and that she would ignore prompts to feed or change her child. Shamira was disengaged from her baby, and it seemed as if she was testing the limits of what she could "get away with" before CPS workers were called. When Sonia was several months old, a report was made to CPS about Shamira's failure to supervise her child or meet her needs, as Sonia went unfed for hours. When this report was made, Shamira made suicidal statements and alternated between begging the authorities not to remove her child and stating that her child would be better off being adopted than with her. Shamira lost custody of Sonia; however, she was allowed to remain in the cottage with Shamira while the baby was in the legal custody of the local department of social services, in hopes that Shamira would be able to improve her parenting skills.

Shamira in the Mommy and Me Group

Throughout this tumultuous time, Shamira consistently attended the Mommy and Me group with Sonia. For the first few months, Shamira remained firmly in the phase of "suspicion and apprehension." Her uncertainty and uneasiness were compounded by the report to CPS, and she expressed the feeling that her parenting was continually being scrutinized. She also voiced the belief that we were "in cahoots" with CPS, and that we would use the Mommy and Me group to glean evidence to ensure that Sonia would be permanently removed from her care. Such a sentiment was understandable, particularly given the profound impact that CPS involvement had had on her own life. During these group sessions, Shamira would sit in an armchair or on the couch, refusing to make eye contact, engage in the group discussions, or interact with Sonia. She would hold Sonia stiffly, often refusing to take off the baby's coat or hat.

As the group progressed into the "tentative exploration" phase, Shamira observed her peers as they began to place their babies on the soft play mat and cautiously interact with the babies and one another. She remained an observer, though. When we gently suggested that perhaps Sonia would enjoy being on the mat with other babies her age, Shamira seemed aghast and stated that she did not think it would be safe for Sonia, since one of the other babies might "hurt her." This assumption was also understandable, given Shamira's own abuse history and subsequent worldview, and served as an important opportunity for education. We explained to Shamira that playful interactions with the mother and other babies are crucial to early child development and positive attachment, and encouraged Shamira to stay close by to keep Sonia safe. She remained unconvinced, and although she would occasionally allow us to hold Sonia for a moment, she interacted minimally with her child and the other group participants.

Shamira's Trauma-Focused Individual Therapy

The watershed moment in Shamira's journey occurred shortly after she began the process of regaining custody of her daughter. In between myriad court appearances, meetings with her court-appointed attorney, and conferences with the local department of social services, Shamira continued to attend weekly individual sessions with me (Stephanie Carnes). During one such session, I observed that Shamira seemed angrier and more distant than usual. With tears in her eyes, Shamira began to describe why the process of CPS involvement was painful and overwhelming. In barely more than a whisper, Shamira explained that she always worried that she would be like her parents, and that the possible removal of her daughter seemed to confirm her fears. While she was adamant that she could not allow her daughter to experience the pain that she had endured as a child, she seemed convinced that the mistakes she had made early in her daughter's life were not the results of her own abuse history, but instead proof that she would be "just like" her parents. She explained that she would not be able to forgive herself if her child grew up in foster care, just as she had after being removed from her parents.

Surprisingly, Shamira subsequently voiced a willingness to explore her own attachment trauma in her individual therapy sessions. With much encouragement from me, Shamira began to speak about her experiences of growing up in an abusive, punitive, and tumultuous household. Several weeks of individual sessions were spent discussing the effects of Shamira's childhood trauma on her development and interpersonal relationships. Like Jamie, Shamira seemed relieved to learn that her symptoms—depression, low self-esteem, shame, guilt, and mistrust of others—were not simply loosely grouped concerns related to organic mental illness, but were instead directly related to the abuse and neglect she had endured through no fault of her own. She and I also focused on her tendency to "zone out" or dissociate. Although this is a common hallmark of attachment trauma, it poses significant challenges, especially to a young mother tasked with caring for a newborn. Shamira was able to identify triggers to her dissociative episodes (such as when her baby's father acted in a controlling, critical manner that reminded her of her own father), and she worked to implement coping skills so that she, in her own words, wouldn't "take it out on Sonia" by ignoring her.

This exploration of Shamira's childhood experiences proved transformative, and the therapeutic work on the effects of her own ruptured attachment and abuse laid the foundation for exploring and understanding her relationship with her daughter. As Shamira began to explore the connection between the abuse she had endured and her current difficulties in engaging with her own child, she seemed almost relieved to learn that she was not deficient, malevolent, or even a bad parent. She was simply reeling from the myriad effects of the most insidious forms of complex childhood trauma. She and I spoke about the differences between meeting her child's needs and nurturing her, and Shamira reflected on her own lack of nurturance and love as a child. I focused on the concept of discipline with Shamira, and we had many discussions about the difference between "making mistakes" as all children do, and "being bad," as she was led to view herself as a child.

As a result of Shamira's extensive complex trauma history, she embodied the belief that the world was a dangerous, threatening place, and she became panicky when Sonia—a happy, social toddler by this point—began to explore her surroundings. We worked to compare and contrast *Shamira's* pervasive fear and uncertainty of the world around her (as a result of her disorganized attachment in childhood) with *Sonia's* desire to explore as a healthy sign that reflected Shamira's strong bond with her. Sonia's experience of the world was far more positive than Shamira's had been. The notion that Shamira could influence her daughter in such a positive way and provide her with the critical components of attachment necessary for cognitive development, emotional well-being, and positive interpersonal relationships seemed to motivate her. The cottage staff noticed that Shamira was now spending more and more time with Sonia, instead of handing her off to another caregiver. In family court hearings, Shamira began to speak proudly of her work in therapy, explaining to the judge that working on her trauma had initiated her shift from a reluctant, frustrated teen parent to an involved, attuned mother.

In individual therapy sessions, Shamira continued to assess her early relationship with her daughter. The focus of therapeutic work became enhancing Shamira's self-esteem and boosting her sense of capability—both of which are important contributors to resilience (Jordan, 2013)—along with the ongoing trauma work. Shamira was able to forgive herself for and find meaning in the early mistakes she had made in her daughter's life, and she and I worked to recognize and honor her steadfast commitment to her child in spite of all she had been through, as evidenced by the zeal and promptness with which she completed all court-ordered services required to return Sonia to her care. Most recently, Shamira has reported experiencing a sense of empowerment as a result of her struggles as a young mother; she is able to recognize the challenges she faced and celebrate the tremendous progress she has made. In a recent therapy exercise using symbols to convey meaning, Shamira selected a heart to represent Sonia because, in her words, "she's my whole heart."

Changes Evident in the Mommy and Me Group

At about the same time, we began to observe a change in Shamira during Mommy and Me group sessions. Although she still needed some prompting to engage consistently with Sonia, especially after spats with Sonia's father, she seemed more relaxed in the group and began to participate in group discussions. She voiced particularly strong opinions on the subject of intimate-partner violence, and she also seemed to develop a sense of pride in her growth as a parent. In addition, since Sonia was older than most of the other babies in the group, the other young moms began to turn to Shamira for advice on breastfeeding and dealing with new babies. Being helpful to others can have a significant impact on promoting caring and resilience, and this has been observed especially in women (Taylor, 2002). Taylor (2002) has referred to this as the "tend-and-befriend" response. Jordan (2013) explains, "Women respond relationally to stress, they seek connection" (p. 77). We would add that helpfulness to others and utilizing social support networks are central to the fostering of resilience. As Shamira's confidence grew, so too did her willingness to try news ways of engaging with Sonia. She became more receptive to encouragement and suggestions from us, and she began to snuggle, read to, and play with Sonia on a regular basis, much to Sonia's delight.

This progress in individual therapy sessions has carried over into the Mommy and Me group. At the time of this writing, Shamira and Sonia are perhaps the most closely bonded of any mother–child dyad in the program. Sonia is a curious, happy, confident, and affectionate toddler who loves spending time with her mother. Shamira has been able to balance her desire to protect and shield Sonia from danger with her newfound understanding that exploratory play facilitates development and attachment. She allows Sonia to roam the play therapy room in which Mommy and Me sessions are held, and she frequently engages Sonia in age-appropriate play activities such as "playing house," "cooking," or play with stuffed animals. When Shamira's peers in the group ask her why her child is so happy and securely bonded with her, she replies with a smile, "I put her first. I know she has to be my priority." Indeed, she has much to be proud of: Less than a year after her daughter was removed from her care, Shamira was once again awarded full custody of her child.

CONCLUDING COMMENTS

Although rates of teen pregnancy have declined in recent years, a subset of the teen population remains at high risk, due to factors associated with social toxicity (Crenshaw & Garbarino, 2007; Crenshaw & Hardy, 2006; Garbarino, 1999; Wolin & Wolin, 1993). These factors include poverty, general lack of opportunity, frustration in educational pursuits, deficiencies in preventive health care, and spiritual emptiness (Crenshaw, 2008; Garbarino & Crenshaw, 2008), as well as family dysfunction and exposure to violence and trauma, often on a continuing basis. These social-environmental factors influence not only the young women who deliver the babies, but also the largely disenfranchised young men who have impregnated them. These teens experience not only frequent tangible losses (such as death of family members, loss of intact families, loss of a place to live, and removal from home), but often intangible losses such as loss of pride, dignity, dreams, vision, and hope (Hardy & Crenshaw, 2008; Hardy & Laszloffy, 2005). The loss of dreams, hopes, and dignity can crush the spirit of a youth, even a hardy teen with a resilient makeup—particularly if the losses are repeated and ongoing. As some youth have described it, such losses are "the nightmare that never ends."

Given the adversity and challenges faced by the young women described in this chapter, it is a marvel to watch these young mothers playing joyfully with their babies, as we did in a recent Mommy and Me group session. The cheerful noises emanating from both the mothers and the babies as they engaged in their playful interactions with one another were heartwarming to witness because such a happy scene is exactly the vision we had for the young mothers when we began the Mommy and Me group in 2012. We found it deeply moving to see the delight the mothers were taking in their babies as they engaged in playful reciprocal sounds, snuggles, and movements on the blankets on the floor. None of these kinds of playful interactions or empathic cuing and matching between mothers and infants were to be seen in the beginning when the mothers joined the group. The very best they were able to do at the start was to hold the babies in their laps—watching over their babies, but not playfully interacting with them. In the beginning, we observed neither delight in the mothers nor any joyfulness in the babies. Obviously, these observations do not constitute hard data. But what we witnessed, in our view, is a striking testament to the resilience of the human spirit. While no one would or should consider such observations scientific, it is hard to ignore what we see with our own eyes (teen mothers playfully interacting with their babies) and what we hear with our own ears (sounds of delight and joy). Quantitative data are being collected and will eventually allow us to report findings as more mothers and babies pass through our program.

For mental health professionals, it can be scary to be delivering therapy to clients when the safety of infants hangs in the balance. If we were not champions of the belief in resilience in our youth, we would not undertake such work. Although the odds to be overcome are akin to the probability that a high school baseball team could win a series against the New York Yankees, we and our CHP colleagues share a conviction about the positive human potential in our youth if they are guided, nurtured, and supported. We do not believe that there was anything extraordinary about our particular therapeutic interventions, but we do believe strongly that the combined efforts of a therapeutic team, a trauma-informed community, and formal group and individual treatment can lead to greater attachment security in teen mothers with complex trauma who have experienced little or no such security in their developmental years. We believe that the increased attachment security of the mothers increased the quality of their bonding and attachment with their babies, and therefore the attachment security of the babies; our observations in the therapeutic living groups and in the Mommy and Me group support this assertion. These young mothers desperately want their babies to have a better life than they have thus far experienced themselves. We greatly admire and respect the longing of these teen mothers to provide their babies with the nurturing, love, and safety they so sorely missed, and we see this as part of their innate healthy drive toward growth, repair, and healing. We are not naive; we know that these mothers and babies have a long road ahead of them. But we take heart in seeing the delight of the mothers as they play with their babies in joyful ways that were completely absent when we began this program. It has reaffirmed our belief in the resilience of our youth even when faced with extreme—often unthinkable and unutterable—adversity.

REFERENCES

Bailey, H. N., Moran, G., & Pederson, D. R. (2007). Childhood maltreatment, complex trauma symptoms, and unresolved attachment in an at-risk sample of adolescent mothers. *Attachment and Human Development, 9,* 139–161.

Bernier, A., & Dozier, M. (2002). The client–counselor match and the corrective emotional experience: Evidence from interpersonal and attachment research. *Psychotherapy: Theory, Research, Practice, Training, 39*(1), 32–43.

Bloom, S. L. (2000). Creating sanctuary: Healing from systematic abuses of power. *Therapeutic Communities: International Journal for Therapeutic and Supportive Organizations, 21*(2), 67–91.

Bonime, W. (1989). *Collaborative psychoanalysis: Anxiety, depression, dreams, and personality change.* Rutherford, NJ: Fairleigh Dickinson University Press.

Cohen, J., Mannarino, A., & Deblinger, E. (2006). *Treating trauma and traumatic grief in children and adolescents.* New York: Guilford Press.

Cook, A., Spinazzolia, J., Ford, J., Lanktree, C., Blaustein, M., Cloitre, M., et al.. (2005). Complex trauma in children and adolescents. *Psychiatric Annals, 35,* 390–398.

Courtois, C. A., & Ford, J. D. (Eds.). (2009). *Treating complex traumatic stress disorders: An evidence-based guide.* New York: Guilford Press.

Crenshaw, D. A. (2008). Multiple sources of child wounding and paths to healing. In D. A. Crenshaw (Ed.), *Child and adolescent psychotherapy: Wounded spirits and healing paths* (pp. 1–14). Lanham, MD: Jason Aronson.

Crenshaw, D. A. (2011). The play therapist as advocate for children in the court system. *Play Therapy, 6,* 6–9.

Crenshaw, D. A. (2012). Secrets told to Ivy. *Play Therapy, 7,* 6–9.

Crenshaw, D. A. (2014). Advocating for vulnerable children. *Play Therapy, 9,* 20–23.

Crenshaw, D. A., & Garbarino, J. (2008). The hidden dimensions: Unspeakable sorrow and buried human potential. *Journal of Humanistic Psychology, 4*(2), 147–160.

Crenshaw, D. A., & Hardy, K. V. (2006). Understanding and treating the aggression of traumatized children in out-of-home care. In N. B. Webb (Ed.), *Working with traumatized youth in child welfare* (pp. 171–195). New York: Guilford Press.

Crenshaw, D. A., & Kenny-Noziska, S. (2014). Therapeutic presence in play therapy. *International Journal of Play Therapy, 23*(1), 31–43.

Erikson, E. H. (1959). *Identity and the life cycle.* New York: International Universities Press.

Garbarino, J. (1999). *Lost boys: Why our sons turn violent and how we can save them.* New York: Anchor Books.

Garbarino, J. (2010). Reverence for spirituality in the healing process. In D. A. Crenshaw (Ed.), *Reverence in the healing process: Honoring strengths without trivializing suffering* (pp. 41–50). Lanham, MD: Jason Aronson.

Garbarino, J., & Crenshaw, D. A. (2008). Seeking a shelter for the soul: Healing the wounds of spiritually empty children. In D. A. Crenshaw (Ed.), *Child and adolescent psychotherapy: Wounded spirits and healing paths* (pp. 49–62). Lanham, MD: Jason Aronson.

Gaskill, R. L., & Perry, B. D. (2014). The neurobiological power of play: Using the Neurosequential Model of Therapeutics to guide play in the healing process. In C. A. Malchiodi & D. A. Crenshaw (Eds.), *Creative arts and play therapy for attachment problems* (pp. 178–194). New York: Guilford Press.

Gregorowski, C., & Seedat, S. (2013). Addressing childhood trauma in a developmental context. *Journal of Child and Adolescent Mental Health, 25*(2), 105–118.

Goldstein, S., & Brooks, R. B. (2013). Why study resilience? In S. Goldstein & R. B. Brooks (Eds.), *Handbook of resilience in children* (2nd ed., pp. 3–14). New York: Springer.

Grossmann, K., Grossmann, K. E., & Kindler, H. (2005). Early care and the roots of attachment and partnership representations. In K. E. Grossmann, K. Grossmann, & E. Waters (Eds.), *Attachment from infancy to adulthood: The major longitudinal studies* (pp. 98–136). New York: Guilford Press.

Hardy, K. V., & Crenshaw, D. A. (2008). Healing wounds to the spirit camouflaged by rage. In D. A. Crenshaw (Ed.), *Child and adolescent psychotherapy: Wounded spirits and healing paths* (pp. 15–30). Lanham, MD: Jason Aronson.

Hardy, K. V., & Laszloffy, T. (2005). *Teens who hurt: Clinical interventions to break the cycle of adolescent violence.* New York: Guilford Press.

Jordan, J. V. (2013). Relational resilience in girls. In S. Goldstein & R. B. Brooks (Eds.), *Handbook of resilience in children* (2nd ed., pp. 73–86). New York: Springer.

Luthar, S. S., & Zelazo, L. B. (2003). Research on resilience: An integrative review. In S. S. Luthar (Ed.), *Resilience and vulnerability: Adaptation in the context of childhood adversities* (pp. 510–549). Cambridge, UK: Cambridge University Press.

Main, M., Goldwyn, R., & Hesse, E. (2003). *Adult attachment scoring and classification system.* Unpublished manuscript, University of California, Berkeley, CA.

Malchiodi, C. A., & Crenshaw, D. A. (Eds.). (2014). *Creative arts and play therapy for problems of attachment.* New York: Guilford Press.

Prince-Embury, S. (2013). The Resiliency Scales for Children and Adolescents: Constructs, research, and clinical application. In S. Goldstein & R. B. Brooks (Eds.), *Handbook of resilience in children* (2nd ed., pp. 273–289). New York: Springer.

Schore, A. N. (2012). *The science of the art of psychotherapy.* New York: Norton.

Shure, M. B., & Aberson, B. (2013). Enhancing the process of resilience through effective thinking. In S. Goldstein & R. B. Brooks (Eds.), *Handbook of resilience in children* (2nd ed., pp. 481–503). New York: Springer.

Siegel, D. J. (2004). Attachment and self-understanding: Parenting with the brain in mind. *Journal of Prenatal and Perinatal Psychology and Health, 18*(4), 273–285.

Siegel, D. J. (2012). *The developing mind: How relationships and the brain interact to shape who we are* (2nd ed.). New York: Guilford Press.

Siegel, D. J., & Hartzell, M. (2003). *Parenting from the inside out: How a deeper self-understanding can help you raise children who thrive.* New York: Tarcher.

Sroufe, L. A. (2005). Attachment and development: A prospective, longitudinal study from birth to adulthood. *Attachment and Human Development, 7*(4), 349–367.

Stewart, A., Whelan, W. F., & Pendleton, C. (2014). Attachment theory as a road map for play therapists. In In C. A. Malchiodi & D. A. Crenshaw (Eds.), *Creative arts and play therapy for attachment problems* (pp. 35–51). New York: Guilford Press.

Taylor, S. (2002). *The tending instinct: How nurturing is essential to who we are and how we live.* New York: New York Times Books.

van der Kolk, B. A. (2005). Developmental trauma disorder: Toward a rational diagnosis for children with complex trauma histories. *Psychiatric Annals, 35,* 401–408.

Webster, L., & Hackett, R. K. (2007). A comparison of unresolved versus resolved status and its relationship to behaviour in maltreated adolescents. *School Psychology International, 28*(3), 365–378.

Wolin, S. J., & Wolin, S. (1993). *The resilient self: How survivors of troubled families rise above adversity.* New York: Villard Books.

Zeanah, C. H., Scheeringa, N. W., Boris, N. W., Heller, S. S., Smyke, A. T., & Trapani, J. (2004). Reactive attachment disorder in maltreated toddlers. *Child Abuse and Neglect, 28*(8), 877–888.

Chapter 10

Playful Pathways
to a Resilient Mindset

*A Play Journey
to Triumph over Adversity*

CHERIE L. SPEHAR

The idea of "resilience" can be a nebulous concept for many. Often confused with "strengths," "resilience" refers to multiple levels of internal and external competence, as well as to confidence within those same areas (see Brooks & Goldstein, Chapter 1, this volume). Internal areas of confidence include such elements as knowledge, recognition, and acceptance of one's existing skills sets; belief in one's abilities; and confidence in worth and self-valuing tendencies.

This chapter describes a number of resource-based interventions in which play therapy has been merged with other expressive modalities—specifically, journal therapy (Spehar, 2014) and mindfulness-based therapy for adolescents and children. These therapeutic approaches synergistically promote resilience, identifying it as not only an intellectual concept, but a broader and deeper sense of well-being that encompasses mind, body, and spirit. Resilience is then seen simultaneously as an internal recognition of resources, and a "felt sense" of how the holistic experience of internal competence is manifested and witnessed.

INTEGRATING JOURNAL THERAPY, MINDFULNESS, AND PLAY THERAPY

As an integrative play therapist, I often create interventions that balance, wed, and support or enhance important intrinsic wellness and individuation factors, such as a client's natural inclinations, the client's identified areas of joy, and intrapersonal and interpersonal efficacy. With that in mind, I introduce three therapeutic modalities (journal therapy, mindfulness, and mindful self-compassion) that even alone have been shown to support a resilient mindset. Here, I share how I have blended them in the art, science, and practice of an integrative approach.

Journal Therapy

A respectable amount of research has been done on the efficacy and outcomes of journal therapy, a profession in the realm of expressive therapies—particularly a journaling approach often referred to as the "Pennebaker method" (Pennebaker, 2004). These studies have shown that "when people write about emotionally difficult events or feelings for just 20 minutes at a time over three or four days, their immune system functioning increases. Pennebaker's studies indicate that the release offered by writing has a direct impact on the body's capacity to withstand stress and fight off infection and disease" (Adams, 1999). As well, journal therapy is promising because it is accessing not only words, but the sensory experiences of the writing itself and of what is being written about. As Voltaire once said, "Writing is the painting of the voice" (Woolf, 1924). With increasing neuroscientific support for the use of sensory methods to treat trauma and traumatic stress, journal therapy becomes a natural and accessible means for the artistic expression of pain. The words themselves can capture a sensory experience of an emotion, while the aesthetic act of forming them becomes a form of expressive art. Journal therapy and expressive writing also introduce flexibility and choice, and both blend easily with play therapy. For instance, journal therapy using the WOWSA method becomes playful because it brings novelty and fun into the process of writing. WOWSA (Spehar, 2013) is an acronym reminding us that the Way we write, what we journal On, what we write With, the Shape of our writing, and what we write About can all introduce the elements of play.

Mindfulness and Mindful Self-Compassion

"Mindfulness is the capacity to step back from, and observe, and be present with the painful mental content" (Hanson & Buczynski, 2011, p. 12).

Thousands of studies are now available on the brain changes that occur with immediate and cumulative mindfulness practices—specifically, changes in neuroplasticity and in the brain centers that regulate emotion and responses to stress. "MRI studies, SPECT scan studies, and EEG studies confirm the ability of mindfulness practice to change brain structures as well as brain functioning. Studies show improvements in self-regulation, mood, well-being, self-esteem, concentration, sleep, health, addictions, memory and so much more" (Burdick, 2013). All of these factors contribute to a resilient mindset.

Even more specific to resilience is "mindful self-compassion" (MSC; Germer, 2009), an arm of mindfulness practice that is crucial to building and sustaining the capacity to manage and be present with thoughts, feelings, situations, and stressors. Thoughts and emotions that cause harm to identity, sense of self, and sense of presence in the world create a lack of empathy for self and others, which in turn has a negative impact on the capacity for accessing and building resilience. In traumatized populations, and many others, MSC is often absent. Victims have been repeatedly reminded by others of their lack of worth, scolded for their apparent faults, blamed for situations, or propelled into a "trance of unworthiness" (Brach, 2012) that prohibits other interventive strategies from being as effective, simply because these individuals don't even deem themselves worthy of healing. MSC practices offer paths of liberation from these destructive internal forces, while simultaneously cultivating a sense of value, purpose, and worth. Advanced MSC then teaches the extension of these practices to others. I find MSC to be an integral, if not essential, component of resilience-driven care.

A synergistic blend of these promising approaches offers advanced practice options for promoting resilience across internal and external life systems. Complex feelings become clearer, more manageable, and less frightening. Journaling and mindfulness practices (including MSC) are also easily accessible, and their use can be self-paced by each client. This alone stimulates a sense of internal mastery and empowerment.

Resilience is also about recognition and meaning making. Recognition of worth, value, and emotions is a catalyst for healthy emotional management and identity shaping. Mindfulness practices encourage the self to be its own witness for internal dynamics. Journal therapy also requires a sense of gentle focus and awareness, and the journal itself becomes an extended witness for the client. Play therapy, journal therapy, and mindfulness practices all provide means for sensory catharsis, which then aid in creating healthy and healing neural pathways. As well, they offer safe, nonthreatening media within which to grow.

INTEGRATION WITH RESILIENCE THEORY

Mindfulness/MSC and Resilience

The use of mindfulness as a way to promote resilience is a natural extension of using the body and mind as a resource. The very premise of mindfulness cultivates the accessibility and adaptability of the brain and body to respond to stress and trauma in healthier ways. Mindfulness (or mindful brain training) invites loving, compassionate awareness of self and situations so that they can be managed without judgment, with less fear, and with greater hope. As well, "the essence of mindfulness is playfulness," so an inherent kindred therapeutic association exists with play therapy interventions (Goldstein, 2013). Mindful play interventions focus on openness, curiosity, absence of judgment, and receptive expression of self. And because one of the most important components of resilience is the value of self, MSC offers exceptional opportunities for the therapeutic process, with activities that encourage holding oneself and the experiences of mind, body, and heart in kind regard at all times. MSC is an important factor in improving overall self-identity and self-worth, as well as in shifting one's self-definition from "victim" to "survivor" to "thriver"—all significant in cultivating a resilient mindset.

Journal Therapy and Resilience

Journal therapy is firmly based in a resilient framework of living in wellness and joy. As James Pennebaker states, "The science and practice of expressive writing continue to complement one another. Science, which moves very slowly, is finding that many different approaches to expressive writing can improve physical and mental health for people dealing with a wide range of problems" (quoted in Adams, 2013). Journal therapy has profound implications for discovering, accessing, and illuminating a resilient mindset and spirit. It is not merely a means to express pain; expressive and emotive writing actually aids in the sensory release of distressing experiences, while simultaneously accessing the pendulum-like motion of examining this pain at different life points and discovering insight and recognition of strengths.

As Kathleen Adams, a pioneer in the profession of journal therapy, has told me, "One of the reasons why journal therapy helps with resilience is because of the way that writing makes a map. We get to see where we have been [and] where we are now, and if we write in alignment with the protocols of embedding internal resources and look at the future with proactivity, writing helps us create a timeline, a map, and a story that we can go back and revisit" (K. Adams, personal communication,

August 8, 2014). Furthermore, Adams indicates that resilience building is about building success upon success, and that the journal becomes a container to hold the successes.

Built into resilience, as well, is the concept of having a therapeutic witness to a person's story. Meaning making for life events is a significant component to the evolution of a resilient mindset. Adams (personal communication, 2014) speaks to this further, stating that "the resilient spirit is one that can place things in a context, and the silent witnessing offers us the context."

KEY TECHNIQUES AND INTERVENTIONS

As noted previously, the interventive approach taken in the cases to be described later in this chapter was a solid combination of mindfulness-based therapy, play therapy, and journal therapy, all of which have supportive studies demonstrating their efficacy. I have created several techniques blending these three modalities and used each of them with the cases described here. I have structured each of these activities so that the reader will find the practicalities easily, while offering deeper discussion of therapeutic application and benefit, reflection, and advanced options. These techniques have been shared with hundreds of clients in my practice over several years; they are those that have consistently helped clients feel safest and most playful, and that have obtained the most efficacious results.

Of special note is a key component of these interventions, called the "sensitive reflection process" (SRP; Spehar, 2014). Kathleen Adams (2013) has created a set of "reflection write" questions, to be answered after any journal entry. (In journal therapy, completed activities are called "writes.") The aims of these questions are to examine the process, to mindfully consider the writing and its message, and to notice any changes in emotional and mental status. Answering these questions is intended to aid a person in recognition and awareness of self. "When we offer . . . the follow-up reflection piece, we can then harvest the insight . . . to find the answers within us and begin to trust that what we accomplish will actually stay where we put it" (K. Adams, personal communication, August 8, 2014). Furthermore, the reflection process for all interventions is essential for resilience building because "The reflection write offers up opportunities for synthesis, integration, awareness, insight, and self-determination. In my experience it amplifies all other benefits to the writing process" (Adams, 2013).

Expanding upon the "reflection write" procedure, the SRP involves deeper therapeutic reflection upon the activity itself, while also providing an opening for sensory reordering and meaning making. The SRP differs from a debriefing: It is intended to sensitively invite mind–body awareness of emotional and affective movement, deepening insights, unexpected lessons, and growth. The richness and depth of healing dynamics are found in this interventive step, and in my opinion, it provides much of the healing context in the interventions described below. When these interventions are used with clients, therefore, the SRP should not be dismissed or minimized. Furthermore, the SRP is meant not to reflect upon content, but upon the process of what happened during an intervention. It is a mindful practice wherein clients are encouraged to notice the way their activities moved them, insights, discoveries, awarenesses, and applications. It also provides the foundation for identity integration in later work.

Paper Plate Stepping-Stones

Created by: Cherie L. Spehar; based on Adams (1990) and Progoff (1992)

Ages: 8 and up

Materials: Any writing utensil; paper plates.

Purposes: To identify important life events; to assess trauma themes; to release emotional energy; to add kinesthetic layers to a healing story; to honor and celebrate life narratives; and to provide insight into and clarity about events affecting a client's life the most (in past, present, and future expressions).

Steps

1. Engage the client in creating Stepping-stones. Stepping-stones (based on techniques originated by Kathleen Adams and Ira Progoff) are a client's 10 most significant milestone events, listed and described from any of several perspectives (e.g., mind, body, heart, spirit). Each set of Stepping-stones typically begins with "I was born" and ends in how the client sees him-/herself, presently or in the future. A client can begin this activity by listing events in the traditional way (on paper first), or by writing them on the paper plates right away.

2. If your client has opted to list the events on paper first, have the client next transfer them creatively and artistically to the paper plates.

3. In a hallway, or a room with enough space, have the client arrange the paper plates on the floor in chronological order. Then, using the following questions to add dimension, depth, and openings

for healing, invite the client to move, touch, step on, or otherwise connect with each Stepping-stone:

> "What do you notice about your Stepping-stones?"
> "Are there any you wish were not in your lifeline?"
> "Move the ones you wish you didn't have to step on or through."
> "What was the hardest one?"
> "Is there one that brought you joy?"
> "Which ones would you turn over, if you could go back in time?"
> "Which ones were the hardest to walk on or through?"
> "Which Stepping-stone is the most meaningful?"
> "Which were the hardest to move on from?"
> "Show me what it was like to move from this one to this one."
> "Which were the happiest?"
> "Which were the slipperiest?"
> "What would happen if you turned this stone over?"
> "Are there any baby pebbles you would add?"
> "What Stepping-stone do you want to get to next?"

4. Store the paper plates in the therapy room, so that they can be used again and again.

Sensitive Reflection Process

You may utilize the Adams "reflection write" method as described earlier in this chapter, or consider asking the following questions:

> "What was it like to complete this activity?"
> "What was the part of this activity you enjoyed most?"
> "What was the part that challenged you most?"
> "What did you experience inside the deepest part of your heart?"
> "How did you feel before this activity? What is different about the way you feel now?"

Therapeutic Discussion

The Paper Plate Stepping-stones activity adds a range of playful elements to therapy. Not only are clients writing *on* something that is unexpected, but clients of all ages enjoy the movement and visual representation of their life stories. This technique is a way of tackling tough topics that invites gentle recognition of the impact of life experiences, develops empowerment, and visually demonstrates the power of a client's journey. It also has the potential to normalize symptoms or provide clarity about the physical expression of stress.

Bridges and Sticks

Created by: Cherie L. Spehar

Ages: 8 and up

Materials: Wooden sticks (e.g., Popsicle sticks); glue; paper; any writing utensil.

Purposes: To demonstrate movement in the healing process; to visually represent pendulation; to capture the process of using sensory regulation skills; to aid in life narrative construction and in meaning making; and to honor life transitions.

Steps

This intervention is another favorite among my clients. It is helpful at all stages of the healing process and can be used not only to show a transition from one emotional state to another, but, on a broader scale, movement from one life passage to another.

1. Mutually determine with a client what aspect of shift, change, transition, or movement the client would like to work on, celebrate, or strengthen. Common ideas or prompts include the following:

> "A bridge from where you were to where you are now."
> "A bridge from where you are now to where you are going."
> "A bridge from one emotional state to another, such as fear to calm, or anger to peace."
> "A healing journey."
> "An identity shift from victim to survivor to thriver."

2. On the wooden sticks, the client may then write the words, phrases, sentences, or heart narratives that represent this transition.

3. On the paper of the client's choosing, have the client place or glue the sticks into the form of a bridge. Clients will naturally find creative ways of constructing this bridge: Some will be layered with supports underneath; others will be in one single glued line.

Sensitive Reflection Process

Again, you may utilize the Adams "reflection write" method, or consider asking the following questions:

"What did this activity show you about your journey?"

"What was the part of this activity that taught you the most?"

"What was the hardest part of your bridge to cross?"

"What does your bridge have underneath it?"

"What was it like to cross to the other side of your bridge?" (Or if the other side is somewhere the client hasn't traveled yet:) "What do you envision the other side might be like?"

"What part of your bridge did you enjoy building the most?"

"What is the view from this part of your bridge? From this other part?"

"Sometimes we walk back and forth across bridges. If you walked back to this side, what would it feel like? If you were standing back at the beginning, how would you be different now? What would look different?"

"What would it be like to go back and travel across this bridge with your new wisdom? Is there anything you might have done differently? Would you have built your bridge with the same tools?"

"What might I see if I crossed the bridge with you?"

Therapeutic Discussion

The metaphor of the bridge is especially helpful in working with clients who sometimes feel stuck. Not only does it help visually demonstrate movement, but it also normalizes the pendulation process in trauma work. Furthermore, this intervention is highly useful for telling life stories and recognizing change. It also invites a client to notice progress, observe the development of resilience, and make meaning of transformations. Finally, Bridges and Sticks can aid in the integration of life experiences and identity.

Tension and Tangles Tamer

Created by: Cherie L. Spehar

Ages: 8 and up

Materials: Journal or writing paper; any writing utensil.

Purposes: To demonstrate movement in the healing process; to visually represent pendulation; to capture the process of using sensory regulation skills; to aid in life narrative construction and meaning making; to honor life transitions; and to teach mindfulness.

Steps

1. Using the concept of poesis, or visual journaling, encourage the client to pick something that feels tangled in his/her life right now.

2. Ask the client to begin the write at the top of the page, using the entire width of the paper, by overlapping the first several sentences so that these visually create a tangle of words.

3. As the client gradually moves to the bottom of the paper, have him/her decrease the width of each line, reduce the number of overlapping words, and add vertical and horizontal space to the words.

4. As this happens, remind the client to write about how the knots are being undone, visually representing the transitional state from tangled to smooth, chaos to calm, emotional dysregulation to tranquility.

5. The end of the write should reach the bottom of the page, and should consist of only one word representing the opposite of the beginning tangle—the concrete symbol of tension being tamed.

Sensitive Reflection Process

Again, you may utilize the Adams "reflection write" method, or consider asking the following questions:

"What did you notice in your body and mind as you completed this write?"

"What do you respond to as you gaze upon your creation?"

"What energy shifts do you notice in the symbols formed by your tangles?"

"Tell me about the energy you feel when you look at your tangles."

"Place your finger on the last word at the bottom of your write. What does it mean to you?"

"With your finger on the last word of your write, try closing your eyes and breathing in the calm of that word, releasing any final tensions as you exhale."

Therapeutic Discussion

Although the Tension and Tangles Tamer is a seemingly simple activity, it holds such energy that clients ask to return to it often for the regulation process. The visual representation of a tense, stressful, or chaotic state of mind and heart becoming calm or untangled is a powerful mechanism to support a mindful approach to stress reduction. Because the activity involves using shapes and writing in a way that is unusual, this introduces the element of play. It is a unique approach to writing in which clients can exercise their artistic brain regions, while simultaneously empowering themselves to undo their emotional, mental, and physical knots in response to stress. As well, this is an activity that can be done easily outside sessions and used as a tool in ongoing practice at home.

Playing in the RAIN

Created by: Cherie L. Spehar; based on Brach (2012)

Ages: 8 and up

Materials: Umbrella; watering can; journal or writing paper; any writing utensil.

Purposes: To teach mindfulness-based stress reduction; to assist in regulating reactions to thoughts and feelings; to create a sense of empowerment and mastery; to help clients make friends with feelings and reduce negative energy from thoughts; and to create pathways of resilience.

Steps

This technique is based on a mindfulness approach developed by Tara Brach; the RAIN acronym is hers. The element of play therapy is added with a prop-based intervention approach.

1. Using the concept of mindful awareness, encourage a client to choose a thought or a feeling the client finds particularly challenging at this time, or one that creates a reaction the client finds uncomfortable.

2. Provide psychoeducation about the concept of RAIN. It may be helpful to start with a mindful awareness practice emphasizing that thoughts are not facts. Then teach the client the art of approaching each part of this thought or feeling, using the acronym RAIN.

  R: Recognizing the thought or feeling, and what is happening in the present moment.
  A: Acknowledging, allowing, and accepting the sensations.
  I: Investigating with intimate attention.
  N: Nonidentification with the thought/feeling (or Nonjudgment of it).

3. Once the concept of RAIN has been playfully introduced, proceed to create a sensory experience of the concept by demonstrating to

the client how RAIN actually creates an umbrella under which to experience the emotions as an observer. (Do this in a location where water can be used.)

4. Using a watering can, gently pour water over an umbrella. Encourage the client simply to notice the "raindrops." Connect the concepts of noticing and being aware of our feelings now as raindrops that pass over us. We can notice them, but not be drenched by them.

5. When this part of the activity is complete, return to the therapy room and have the client complete a "process write" (a journal therapy narrative) of what he/she wishes to remember about feelings, thoughts, and using RAIN.

Sensitive Reflection Process

Again, you may utilize the Adams "reflection write" method, or consider asking the following questions:

> "What did you notice in your body and mind as you completed this activity?"
> "What is it like to learn that thoughts are not facts?"
> "What is the part of RAIN that might be hardest for you? Easiest?"
> "What do you think you will remember most about this activity?"
> "How has what you learned or experienced with this activity help you?"
> "Which part was the most fun? Why?"

Therapeutic Discussion

Playing in the RAIN is a practical and accessible tool for enabling clients to work with stressful thoughts and feelings in a nonjudgmental and compassionate way. Because we do not judge a feeling or thought as good–bad, rational–irrational, or positive–negative, we can teach clients to accept it as it is. It is particularly important to note that acceptance does not mean approval. This distinction is often necessary because reactions to thoughts and feelings can be unsettling, and we do not want clients to think they are being asked to like them/approve of them. Rather, we are simply accepting that the thoughts and feelings exist.

Finally, this tool is an excellent way to encourage MSC, which, as described earlier in this chapter, is key to building internal resilience and care. Goldstein (2013) states about RAIN that this practice encourages emotional freedom and aids clients in making friends with feelings. It is a strengths-based approach to emotion regulation and distress tolerance.

My Heart, Your Heart

Created by: Cherie L. Spehar; based on Catlin (personal communication, April 19, 2013)

Ages: 8 and up

Materials: None.

Purposes: To enhance empathy for self and others; to foster a sense of connection and belongingness; to facilitate the practice of mindfulness and MSC; and to foster resilience.

Steps

This intervention involves more of the meditative aspects of mindfulness and MSC. It is an excellent activity to use with groups and families, as well as for individual work.

1. Begin by describing the nature of an imagery activity, and gently invite the client or clients to a unique experience in which they will be able to experience the potential for stillness, connection, and peace.

2. Once clients are oriented to the nature of the activity, begin by taking them outside and asking them to take their shoes off and stand on a part of the earth. This should be sand, grass, dirt, or some other natural part of the earth (not concrete, brick, wood, etc.).

3. Ask clients to close their eyes and notice the feel of the earth beneath them. Then follow this script:

> "As you notice your feet touching the earth, what do you feel? Is it soft? Cold? Warm? Do you notice the grass tickling or itching? What else do you notice about the way the earth touches your body?"
>
> "Next, begin to notice the way you are breathing. One of the most important parts of reaching stillness is to breathe with intention. Exhale deeply to release all of your tension. Take a few deep breaths in and out, and notice the earth speaking to you."
>
> "As you breathe deeply, I want you to place a hand on your heart and notice its rhythm. Is it fast? What sound does it make in your head? What does your hand notice as you feel your heart drumming beneath your fingers?"
>
> "Next, notice what your heart is saying in those beats. Perhaps there is a longing or a sadness. Maybe it is telling you it is

weary and uncertain. Listen to the message of your heart, and stay quietly with that a moment."

"Now come back to your feet. Realize that at this moment—whatever you are experiencing, and whatever you are feeling—the very earth, the very planet beneath you, is supporting you. The earth is tending to you and letting you know that if you fall, it will catch you. Feel the energy of the earth reaching up to tend to your feet and send you a message right into your core."

"As you contemplate this awareness, let it come to you that perhaps at this very moment, another person directly on the other side of the world has stopped and is standing with bare feet upon this same earth. And in this moment, you make a connection to that person's energy. Tune in to the person you may be connected to, this very moment. Breathe in, breathe out. Recognize that you are not alone, and that your earth partner on the other side of the world may be extending energy to you at this very moment."

"Keeping your hand on your heart, say to your heart, 'My heart, may you be calm. My heart, may you be rested. My heart, may you be soothed.' And to the person on the other side of the world, extend compassion and kindness: 'Friend, may you feel belonging. Friend, may you feel safe. Friend, may you feel supported.'"

"As you complete this blessing, come back with knowing that you are not alone, and that you have held your heart and another's in loving kindness. Breathe in, and then do a long exhale. Another. When you are ready, open your eyes."

"When you have come back to this place, consider taking a moment to write down some thoughts and feelings about your experience."

4. Provide ample time for clients to sit outside (or come to a safe and warm space inside) and write down the nature of their experience.

Sensitive Reflection Process

Reflection questions for a meditative process should focus on the nature of the experience. Some clients may wish to share what they saw, or whom they imagined, and this is fine. If clients are reflecting in a group, try to make space for this without pressure to do so. To facilitate the SRP, you may wish to try the following prompts:

"What did you notice about the feel of the earth?"

"What was it like for your body to actually touch the living planet?"

"What would you like to share about the idea of connecting to someone on the other side of the world?"

"What happened when you really paid attention to your breathing?"

"What sensations came up for you when you imagined not being alone in the world?"

"If you could have said something to your earth companion, what might you have said?"

"What was your favorite part of this activity?"

"What did this activity help you with?"

"How do you think you might return to this activity, or parts of it?"

Therapeutic Discussion

Feeling less alone and having a sense of belonging are vital and tangible expressions of resilience. Trust in the knowledge that we are seen, heard, and understood is the basis of relational health. "If you want to build up the neural substrate of these very comforting, soothing attachment circuits, that are deeply woven into the fabric of our being . . . then you are going to call to mind and encourage clients to call to mind the sense of being cared about" (Hanson & Buczynski, 2011, p. 15).

Fused

Created by: Cherie L. Spehar (Spehar, 2011)

Ages: 8 and up for children, and any age for adults (parents/other caregivers)

Materials: None, or a blanket if child prefers.

Purposes: To enhance parent/caregiver–child connections; to teach mindfulness, distress tolerance, sensory soothing; to build resilience and support posttraumatic growth; and to activate natural healing instincts (to create a positive "fusion" between children and their trusted adults).

Steps

This intervention was created several years ago to aid parents (or other caregivers) in facilitating a sensory experience of safety, soothing, and support. Often the missing link in doing so is tuning in to the felt sense of words and actions. This is an activity that can be broadened and generalized to multiple parent–child interactions.

1. *Freeze.* Ask parents to "freeze" and notice as much as possible about their own sense of awareness in the moment. Self-assessment is vital before a parent can genuinely attune to a traumatized child.

2. *Undivided attention umbrella.* Now ask each parent to release other distractions, focusing completely on the child. Have the parent tell the child, "Guess what! It's invisible umbrella time! We are under our invisible umbrella shelter, and you and I are super-safe under here together! How can we fit under here? Let's snuggle! What does it feel like under here?"

3. *Sensory synergy.* This step is where the magic happens. Encourage each parent to "snuggle" with the child under the invisible umbrella in a way that promotes sensory safety—for example, "Hold Mommy's hands and feel how warm they are!" Have the parents help the children tune in to the physical sensation of closeness, warmth, and safety. Use sensory language. Ask the children to notice the felt experience of being held.

4. *Express and expand.* Have parents ask children how they can take this safe and special feeling with them. Have them find words together that engage the brain at the instinctual level.

5. *Delight demonstration.* Traumatized children need *noticing.* In this step, each parent demonstrates absolute delight in the child and the experience by using words and physical affection simultaneously.

Sensitive Reflection Process

As always, you may utilize the Adams "reflection write" method, or consider asking the following questions. (In addition, one of the best ways to reflect upon this process and sensation is to have all involved draw a picture of what it felt like.)

"What was the best feeling you had in your snuggle space?"
(For children:) "What did you like most about what your mom/dad/ caregiver said or did?"
"What parts felt different or unusual?" (This is an important SRP question, as an important aim of this exercise is to create as comfortable a process as possible. This will mean understanding the family members' energy, how they respond to one another,

and helping them find their specific language to make this activity come alive in the best way for their family culture.)

"Write down one feeling word about what this was like for you."

(For children:) "Write a message to your mom/dad/caregiver about what you enjoyed about this activity."

(For parents/caregivers:) "Write a message to your child about what was special about this activity. How did you find delight in the child and the experience?"

Therapeutic Discussion

Fusion is a simple but powerful connective technique to help parents and other caregivers become therapeutic healing agents. By creating space for regular, consistent, and fun "meaning moments"—concentrated doses of undivided, mutually intrinsic, delighted attention—it provides a chance for children to experience sensations of grounding and empowerment, while also amplifying the child–parent connection. Because it feels unrushed, because it is anchored in a sensory experience, and because both children and adults are active participants, healing is influenced on multiple levels, therefore building resilience and supporting posttraumatic growth.

Partnership Pledge Circle

Created by: Cherie L. Spehar

Ages: Family members (or other persons close to a family) of all ages

Materials: A large sheet of paper (16 × 20 inches) for each family; a variety of art supplies.

Purposes: A wise mentor, Teresa Illinitch, once taught me, "People tend to support that which they themselves create." As I have found this to be at least anecdotally true across systems and practices, the purposes of this activity are to encourage ownership of the healing process and family unity; to help family members recognize their support of one another, and thus to support a resilient family mindset; to enhance a family's internal and external resources; and to offer family members a tool for accessing stability and safety outside the professional setting, which is where the most growth will occur.

Steps

1. Introduce the activity by explaining that we are all partners in the process of healing—from those closest to a child client, moving

outward in stages of connection and acquaintance. Family, friends, coaches, teachers, extended kin, and other trusted adults can all be part of this exercise.

2. On a large piece of paper, have participants draw a circle that will become the Partnership Pledge Circle.

3. Within the circle, have participants draw as many hearts as there are family members. This can be done in any fashion. Some draw the hearts so that bottom points of the hearts all touch in the center; others just draw random hearts within the circle.

4. Have each person present select a heart. Ask each person to draw a line through the middle of his/her heart. Say: "In one half of your heart, write a way in which you will give yourself compassion and kindness. In the other side, write how you will show the same toward others in this family system."

5. Ask all family members to engage in decorating their Partner Pledge Mandala with whatever art supplies are desired.

6. When the Partnership Pledge Circle is complete, make space for clients to read their writing aloud. If they choose not to do so, family members can read the writing in silence.

Sensitive Reflection Process

As always, you may utilize the Adams "reflection write" method, or consider asking each person in the group the following questions:

"Please write down at least three things you experienced about the process or about what was shared."

"Notice your Partnership Pledge Circle. What do you see? What energy does it bring you?"

"What themes are present with your family voice?"

"If your Partnership Pledge Circle was hanging in a museum or gallery, what would people say about it?"

"What does this activity mean to you?"

"What did you notice about what your other family members said?"

"What feelings came up for you when you heard how other family members pledged their compassion and kindness?"

"What impact do you think this might have on your life after you leave today?"

"What do you hope might be different for your family?"

"What does your body feel like after sharing this experience with your family?"

Therapeutic Discussion

Circles or mandalas are tools I frequently use in combination with journal therapy. Symbolically, they are rich with meanings of unity, completeness, and wholeness. In work to foster a sense of partnership and continuity in a family or extended system, a circle or mandala as a symbol alone helps to create a sense of togetherness. The concrete act of making a pledge within the family mandala not only deepens the experience, but also gives on each member of the system a sense of gentle accountability. Beyond that, family members receive a sense of connection, as well as insight into each other. They are able to see one another's vulnerabilities when the extensions of compassion toward selves are written and heard, while simultaneously witnessing the care they have for one another. The SRP then aids them in giving shape and form to their reactions.

CLINICAL CASE EXAMPLE: MICAH

Vulnerability and Risk Factors

When Micah first came to my office, he was a 13-year-old boy struggling with a number of symptoms related to chronic traumatic stress. Because so many life events had contributed to his symptoms, his vulnerability to continued risk taking, substance use, and traumatic relationships was high. Furthermore, Micah's risk factors were severe. Not only was he at risk for failing his current grade level; he was beginning to engage in behaviors that threatened to place him swiftly in the court system. He ran away from home often, broke into cars to disable their ignitions, and was becoming a "known suspect" in the police system. Micah's struggles did not end there, however. In addition to his traumatic past, his current lifestyle put him at continual risk for drug use, drug running, and gang involvement. Basic survival was a daily "microtrauma," as gunshots were heard outside his home almost every night. Moreover, Micah had few resources in the community with whom or which he felt emotionally safe enough to turn for help. Those individuals who once supported him were beginning to see him as a lost cause; they were becoming increasingly disappointed in his seemingly irrational behaviors and refusal to "listen to reason." They frequently said things to him that perpetuated a cycle of secondary wounding—blaming, minimizing, and shaming him.

Micah's own pain and private logic also created a pattern of internal self-harm called "self-secondary wounding." Far deeper than negative self-talk, this is a belief system mired in hopelessness, deficiency, and permanency.

Protective Factors

However, Micah's behaviors had other messages to give to the world. There was a light within him that was enhanced by a number of factors, as noted from our 40 Developmental Assets assessment of him (Search Institute, n.d.). For one thing, Micah had a deep and abiding connection to a sense of existential "otherness." He did not feel as if he could identify what God meant to him, but he was able to say that he did not feel spiritually alone, though he often had trouble finding his spiritual feeling. Along with this, Micah had an innate sense of humor that invited all to smile with him. Although he often used humor as a distractor or a defense, Micah still amazed people with his ability to smile at all.

Challenges and Adversity

As noted above, Micah's trauma history was significant. He came from a home that was rife with emotional, mental, and physical chaos. Daily, he witnessed physically and verbally violent exchanges between his mother and father, and he was also continually threatened with abandonment by both parents. One evening, after a particularly brutal exchange, his father left the house and said he was never coming back. Later he was found dead, a suicide; the teenagers who found him then sent Micah pictures of his dead body. Micah's relationship with his mother grew even worse after this, as she blamed him for his father's death. Not surprisingly, Micah's grades plummeted; he began to run away from home and stay out all night; and he started looking for other peers with whom he could feel accepted. Micah was exposed to many gang invitations, and began some initiation processes with two gangs before he was brought to my care and attention.

The Shift to a Resilient Mindset

Micah was one of the most initially subdued clients I had ever seen. His internal struggle was visibly present: His desire to trust was constantly at war with his fear of what would happen if he did. The interventions that helped Micah begin to identify his world as less hostile began with basic mindful awareness practices, and one of the most powerful moments occurred when he resonated with the idea that "thoughts are not facts." Playfully, we began a scientific exploration of his thoughts, forming hypotheses and theories about them. Ultimately, Micah conceded that there was no way to prove a thought. This set the stage for the realization that part of the process of finding his way in the world would be to address his private logic and belief systems, so that every worried, upset, or damaging thought he had would not be perceived as a fact. When Micah started to integrate this idea into his everyday life, a shift began: He started to see less trauma lurking everywhere, and more positive potential.

Once Micah began achieving some degree of sensory regulation through his new insights, he was even more receptive to exploring (via the interventions noted below) his life events—both the negative ones that had traumatized him, and the positive ones that had given rise to the rudimentary belief system he had. In the Paper Plate Stepping-stones exercise (described earlier in this chapter), Micah could visually see that there were many reasons for his life to feel chaotic, unstable, and unsafe. However, his reflections about his Stepping-stones also shifted his focus to the massive amounts of strength he had shown to overcome so much trauma and still smile.

Once Micah began moving through the basics of understanding his life and how it had shaped him, he became an avid listener and willing participant in therapy. Although he was still sullen on some days, he enjoyed play-based journal therapy activities because these offered him time to be quietly introspective without pressure, in the presence of a trusted adult.

Following is a snapshot of one of his activities, the Tension and Tangles Tamer (also described earlier in this chapter).

MICAH: I don't feel like talking today, Ms. S. I'm doing my MAPs [mindful awareness practices], but FML [slang abbreviation for "f*** my life"] right now. My mom called.

THERAPIST: You've taught me about this feeling for you. That usually means there is something you still want to come out but not talk about it. Am I reading that right today?

MICAH: Yeah. I just need to do it. [This was important because Micah was recognizing the value in something that had worked for him before and was asking for it now.]

THERAPIST: I have some new ideas for you with writing, or you could pick one you've already tried.

MICAH: Yeah. I need to do that one where you undo the knots.

THERAPIST: The Tension and Tangles Tamer? All right, let's give it a go. (*Sets up all materials.*) [I was allowing selection and choice for Micah in how he wanted to create his Tension and Tangles Tamer. This was an intervention with which he was familiar, and he needed little further instruction.]

MICAH: (*Beginning to write*) And so I don't need to tell you everything she said. I can just twist it all up at the top with, like, what it feels like and the shit she said.

THERAPIST: Yes, that's exactly right. Would you like some music, or just silence?

MICAH: I don't know—like, that stuff where it just sounds like a flute or something would be OK. I mean, it's not the music I like or anything, but I like it in here.

THERAPIST: (*Sets up Native American flute music as per Micah's previous selections.*)

Micah then began to write, while I sat in reverence and quietly observed. The intention of a therapist's being present in an intervention like this is to be connected and available, but not to hover over the client or monitor every detail, as this will create an element of discomfort. At this time, the therapist can jot down some reflections on the client's posture and other physical indicators (the way the pen is being held, shifts in emotional energy, breathing, the places where the client's tension appears to be held in the body, etc.). After Micah reached the point where he felt he had completed his write, the SRP began.

THERAPIST: So. Let's take a breath. I noticed things changing for you, things like your posture and your breathing while you were writing. . . . What happened during this write?

MICAH: I didn't really want to do it at first, but I mean—I don't know, I knew I had to, 'cause there was poison in me.

THERAPIST: You had to write. That's a pretty important piece of knowing . . . your wisdom inside you was speaking. What happened to the poison as you wrote? [Notice that I did not seek specifics about the poison; I allowed that to unfold on its own if Micah chose to share.]

MICAH: Well, I was diluting it. Like in chemistry. By the time I got to the bottom, I feel like the poison isn't in me anymore; it's in her.

THERAPIST: I think I'm following you. . . . What does that mean for you?

MICAH: Like (*pause, eyes misting*), it helps me see that first I can calm down. But really, Miss, like we been sayin' . . . it shows me that even though she can pour poison on me and in me, and I came from her poison, I don't have to keep it. [Notice the resilient mindset that Micah was accessing and also creating in the moment. Also, consider that he and I did not need to spend time talking about everything the poison meant. He had already regulated his emotional state with the intervention, and further processing of content was not necessary.]

THERAPIST: I feel the power with you of what you are saying and sharing. What is happening for you in this moment?

MICAH: It's like, this is the first time I didn't go all 911, ya know? Like all the other times when she, like, called me or on home visits, I wanna die or somethin'. This time there was somethin' I could do. But I still wanted to come here to try it. [Micah enjoyed the safe haven of the therapy room, and often spoke of feeling calm and protected there. It was especially powerful that he wanted to practice this activity on his own, while still recognizing that he felt the pull toward an anchoring space to do so.] Guess I'm talkin' now, huh? (*Smiles.*)

THERAPIST: You are indeed. Is this kind of talking OK?

MICAH: Yeah, like we're not even talkin' about all the shit she said. We just showin' me I'm strong.

THERAPIST: I'm really honored to walk this with you. I wonder if we could try the last part of this activity . . . where you place your finger on the last word, the calmer word, and tell me what it means to you? (*Thoughtfully, Micah does so.*)

MICAH: Miss . . . I don't know if this is a word or somethin' for a feeling. But when I look at the top and then the bottom, it's just, like, it's all good.

Subsequent revisits of this particular intervention further aided Micah in recognizing his inherent strengths, as well as providing him with a mechanism to reframe the emotional dysregulation that conversations with his mother often elicited. His SRP accounts are, to this day, some of the most moving I have ever witnessed.

Micah also had significant difficulty in showing empathy to others because he had little to none for himself. With MSC exercises (which he initially called "those crazy trips"), Micah allowed his heart to soften to himself, and in turn to others. After the My Heart, Your Heart exercise (also described earlier in this chapter), Micah allowed me to see his tears for the first time. He said, "I know you are with me. And I know someone else, somewhere, is too." Although it did not happen immediately after this session, Micah soon became a group volunteer at his placement setting, to help others learn to care enough about themselves not to hurt themselves or others.

Community support was very important to Micah's reordering and recovery. As noted earlier, Micah had often experienced secondary wounding from other trusted adults, and it took a long time for him to trust some key adults not to hurt him. I was privileged to be one of them. Because of the gift of trust he ultimately gave me, he walked with me—and eventually others—through exercises designed to promote connection and belonging. In the Partnership Pledge Circle exercise, for example, Micah included me, his basketball coach, and his music director, along with his mother, aunt, grandmother, and brother. I would like to share some portions of the SRP that followed this exercise, to demonstrate the healing that occurred. For brevity, I focus primarily on the reflections of Micah and his mother.

> THERAPIST: Wow . . . I know that I am feeling like I've just witnessed something just amazing. There's a lot of energy in this room right now; do you feel it? Now that we have all participated in the Partnership Pledge Circle, let's take a minute to collect our thoughts and consider all that was shared. Maybe let's all jot down a few words or thoughts or feelings as we sit together in silence. [This is part of a capturing concept used in journal therapy. It blends mindful awareness with reflection, and participants usually take no more than a minute or two to complete it and gather themselves for the larger reflection.]
>
> THERAPIST: What does this activity mean to you?
>
> MICAH: I'm sayin', I never knew that people cared so much like the way you said it here. And I never thought I would be coloring stuff with people who cared. (*The group laughs.*)
>
> MOTHER: I don't know what to say. I messed up all the way. But this, here today . . . I guess what it means is a start.
>
> THERAPIST: Mmm. I can see the power in what is happening, yes. What did you notice about what your other family members said? What stood out the most for you?
>
> MOTHER: I guess for me, it was watching Micah have to write about how he won't hurt himself. 'Cause really I'm the reason for that, and . . . it's hard to swallow. But I look around this room (*crying now*), and know I have a long way to go, but I have such love in my heart that God saw to it to watch over my boy with y'all.
>
> MICAH: I'm sayin' . . . just thank you.

THERAPIST: It will be time to wrap up soon and carry this with you once you leave this room. What impact do you think this might have on your life after you leave today?

MICAH: Man, Miss, you askin' all the questions that get those onions in my eyes. [This was a reference to a previous joke: At first Micah didn't want to call his tears, when they appeared, "tears." The term "onions" was his way of using humor, and of softening what was happening when he was filled with emotion.] But, for real, this is a'right. These the people I can count on. So, yeah. That's what I'm takin' with me.

MOTHER: For the future? This is my reminder. My reminder to do good. To serve God. To serve him by loving my son right.

After Micah made this journey from the smallest of steps to the point of recognizing his own strength, using it to help himself and others, and reordering his experience in his own way and at his own pace, he was finally able to make the transition to independent living. Shortly before that happened, I left for another state, and so I was not able to continue with him on the final part of his supported path.

About 3 years later, Micah located me professionally and sent an email to my website address. One paragraph read:

I don't know how you did what you did. I don't know how I did what I did. But what I do know is that somehow I like who I am now. And I like that you helped me find me. (Don't I sound like I am writing a poem? You always said that to me!) Anyway, I know I can do anything now.

CONCLUDING COMMENTS

Incorporated into the practices described in this chapter are additional tools the reader may choose to assess and foster resilience. Although not specifically mentioned as part of the interventive methods, they are relevant to broadening clinical perspectives on resilience. To that end, my recommendations for further information and reading would include the 40 Developmental Assets framework developed by the Search Institute (n.d.) and the concept of "multiple intelligences" championed by Howard Gardner (e.g., Gardner, 2006). The Search Institute provides the reader with a comprehensive guide to and checklists of research-based conditions across all age groups that have been found in resilient children and adults, with some ideas on how to enhance them. Embracing the multiple-intelligences concept involves asking not "Is this person smart?" but "How is this person smart?" I have incorporated these tools into my practice for more than 15 years, and they provide assistance for clinicians, clients, families, and extended community systems in learning not only how to recognize inherent and natural resources, but how to reach individuals in the places where their internal capacities come alive.

The practices highlighted in this chapter are designed to demonstrate a synthesis of playful interventions enhanced by other effective methods for furthering resilience.

Resilience-focused practices are essential in work to help child clients overcome adversity. Working from a resource-based model of care, clients develop a greater capacity for joy, as well as the potential for evolving to activate the best version of themselves at any given point in their lives. It should also be stated that involving parents/trusted adults as healers in the process, even if they have shared the same traumas as their children, offers benefits across family systems that can enhance their mutual recovery and strengthen family identity. It answers the children's need for assurances that their caregivers *see* them. And most significantly, the simple miracle of family members' sharing the most powerful healing agents of all—themselves—is a demonstration of resilience.

Finally, a key aspect of cultivating resilience is the shaping and reshaping, forming and reforming of resourceful identities. Going far deeper than self-esteem, a resourceful identity is one that embodies the characteristics not only of a survivor, but of a thriver. Surviving offers a sense of accomplishment, bravery, and pride at having made it through the most challenging circumstances imaginable; moving into thriving propels individuals into a state of being where resilience shines. It is characterized by positive risk taking; immersion and enjoyment in life; comfort with the unknown; open and flexible thinking; and a consistently compassionate response to self and others. Our responsibility as privileged practitioners in a healing role is to facilitate the recognition, awareness, growth, and sustainability of this internal and external state. A thriving mindset will serve as the substrate for all of life's steppingstones to come.

REFERENCES

Adams, K. (1990). *Journal to the self: 22 paths to personal growth.* New York: Warner Books.

Adams, K. (1999). A brief history of journal writing. Retrieved January 27, 2013, from *http://journaltherapy.com/journaltherapy/journal-to-the-self/journal-writing-history*

Adams, K. (2013). *Expressive writing: Foundations of practice.* Lanham, MD: Rowman & Littlefield Education.

Brach, T. (2012). *True refuge: Finding peace and freedom in your own awakened heart.* New York: Bantam Books.

Brach, T. (n.d.). Working with difficulties: The blessings of RAIN. Retrieved June 4, 2013, from *www.tarabrach.com/articles/RAIN-WorkingWithDifficulties.html*

Burdick, D. (2013). *Mindfulness skills workbook for clinicians and clients: 111 tools, techniques, activities and worksheets.* Eau Claire, WI: Pesi.

Gardner, H. (2006). *Multiple intelligences: New horizons* (rev. ed.). New York: Basic Books.

Germer, C. K. (2009). *The mindful path to self-compassion: Freeing yourself from destructive thoughts and emotions.* New York: Guilford Press.

Goldstein, E. (2012). *The now effect: How this moment can change the rest of your life.* New York: Atria Books.

Goldstein, E. (2013, June 19). 3 key mindfulness practices for calm, self-compassion and happiness [Web log post]. Retrieved from *http://blogs.psychcentral.com/mindfulness/2013/06/3-key-mindfulness-practices-to-feel-happy-and-free.*

Hanson, R., & Buczynski, R. (2011, September 30). Neurodharma: How to train the brain toward mindfulness. Retrieved October 29, 2014, from *http://files.nicabm.com/Mindfulness2012/pre-series/hanson/Rick_Hanson.pdf.*

Pennebaker, J. W. (2004). *Writing to heal: A guided journal for recovering from trauma and emotional upheaval.* Oakland, CA: New Harbinger.

Progoff, I. (1992). *At a journal workshop: Writing to access the power of the unconscious and evoke creative ability.* Los Angeles: Tarcher.

Search Institute. (n.d.). Developmental assets. Retrieved November 6, 2014, from *www.search-institute.org/research/developmental-assets.*

Siegel, D. (n.d.). Mindfulness, psychotherapy and the brain. Retrieved March 7, 2013, from *www.ithou.org/node/2730.*

Spehar, C. L. (2011, August 23). Creating connections [Web log post]. Retrieved from *http://tlcinstitute.wordpress.com/2011/08/23/creating-connections.*

Spehar, C. L. (2013, October). *The playful path of the pen: Play based journal therapy.* Paper presented at the annual conference of the Association for Play Therapy, Palm Springs, CA.

Spehar, C. L. (2014, April 24). *The playful path of the pen: Play based journal therapy.* Paper presented at annual conference of the Passion to Profit Journal Therapy, Scottsdale, AZ.

Woolf, H. I. (Ed. & Trans.). (1924). *Voltaire's philosophical dictionary.* New York: Knopf.

Index

The letter *f* following a page number indicates figure; the letter *t* indicates table.